You **Tutorial**

Hairstyling

Your guide to the best instructional YouTube videos

CARLTON BOOKS

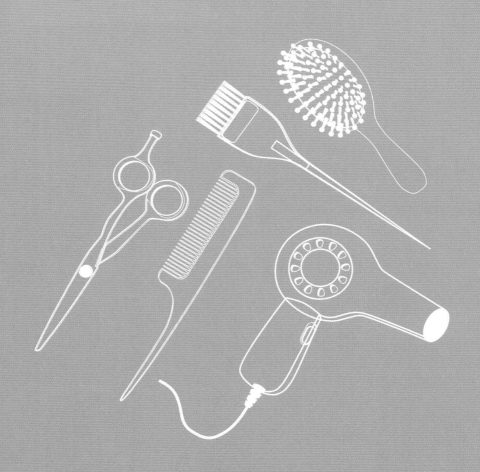

Contents

INTRODUCTION

How to use this book

These days there's a YouTube video tutorial for *everything* – especially when it comes to looking good. In the space of just a few years, the video-sharing site has proved to be the perfect medium for hair and beauty tutorials. Not so long ago, many styles were only ever attempted by hair professionals, but in this YouTube age, any girl with a webcam and a bit of hair know-how can upload a step-by-step video explaining how to recreate a look.

But with such a vast array of hair vlogs out there, all promising to teach you the best way to achieve salon-worthy locks, it's tough to know which clip to click on. That's where this book comes in. If you can't decide which YouTuber is the best stylist or haircare guru

for you, this handy guide will help make life easier. We've carefully selected more than 100 of the best and most popular hair videos ever uploaded to YouTube, so you can find and watch them fast without wasting countless hours trawling the internet.

Want to learn how to create the perfect waterfall braid or the easiest way to get lasting beachy waves? Do you need a straightforward lesson in professional-style blow-drying or perhaps you fancy dyeing your own hair but want to avoid a DIY disaster? Whatever your hair needs, we've got the perfect video for you – right here.

The tutorials in this book are curated from the most successful hair vloggers on the web, with many videos selected because they have achieved the highest number of views on that subject. Plus, you'll also find equally enlightening clips from some lesser-known vloggers – up-and-coming stylists with amazing skills and large personalities that you won't want to miss. We guarantee you'll find a good few new YouTube hair channels to subscribe to along the way.

Each of the reviews explains why the tutorial is a must-see, along with details of the channel and vlogger behind it, and has both a URL address and QR code so you can instantly find and view the real thing.

So, what are you waiting for – more than 100 great new hair looks are just a click away!

How to View the Clips

Each entry is accompanied by a QR code, which you can scan with your digital device using apps such as Quick Scan, QR Reader or ScanLife. Alternatively there is a short URL address which you can type into your browser. Unfortunately the adverts preceding some of the clips are unavoidable but it's usually possible to skip them after a few seconds.

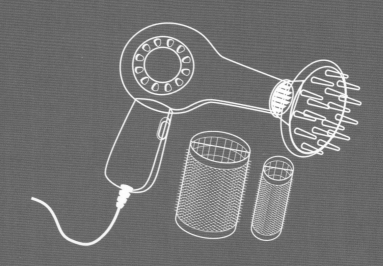

CREATING

Curls and Waves

Speed Curls

Add curls fast
with Elle Fowler

Since 2008, Elle Fowler's beauty tutorials on her YouTube channel AllThatGlitters have had millions of views thanks to her bubbly persona and expert tips. Here she shares her perfect formula for curls in a hurry, including the silky styling gel-mousse she applies to her hair while it's wet to protect it and ensure the curls stay put. Next she grabs a chunky curling tong and demos her easy twist technique for casual loose curls, using large sections of hair. But by far her most useful advice in this tutorial is how to get curls that swirl the right way – out from your face – on both the left and right. It's a detail most of us would never even think of, but it makes all the difference, as Elle proves.

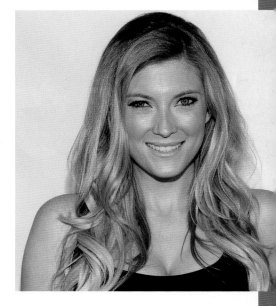

http://youtu.be/pzaNNhHbCJ0

Soft Curls

Blair Fowler's recipe for gentle daily waves

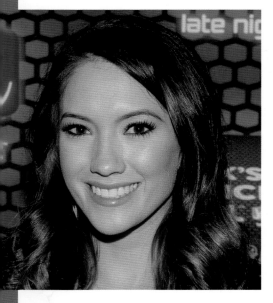

It wasn't long before big sis Elle Fowler got her younger sister Blair into vlogging and she became a go-to makeup guru in her own right with her own much-watched channel Juicystar07. Blair gets many questions from her vlog watchers on her gorgeous wavy brown hair, so she created a video that shows exactly how she styles it. She favours a few drops of hair oil treatment applied while damp and uses an old-fashioned blowdryer until her hair is three-quarters dry. Next it's time to reveal her technique for using hair tongs – notably different from her sister's method. Blair picks a smaller barrel tong and uses it to create tighter, more ringlet-style curls. She then brushes her whole hair out to cleverly soften the look.

http://youtu.be/HSq5p6MLPU8

Wavy Hair – No Heat Required

Weylie's secret for
effort-free waves

Weylie's unique mix of quirky style, cool graphics
and useful advice has drawn more than 1 million
subscribers to her YouTube channel ilikeweylie.
The fun, young vlogger delivers her popular tutorials
in an upbeat, friendly style. Here she shares her
secret for waking up with your hair in waves. The
first step is to wash hair and apply a little leave-in
conditioner when it's still damp. Weylie then shows
how to twist your hair and roll it into a bun secured
by a scrunchie – yes, a scrunchie – before leaving
it overnight. It's hard to believe, but when she takes
the bun out next morning, she's left with a cascade
of perfectly tousled curls – no styling required. A
must-try technique!

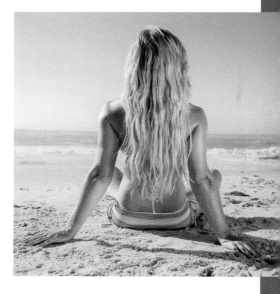

Curl Hair with Straighteners: Long Hair

Learn a cool new tool for curling
with Riannstar

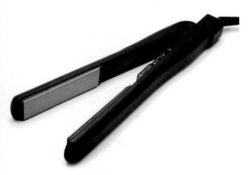

If you've only been using your straightening irons to smooth your locks until they're poker-straight, then you're missing a trick. You can create beautiful ringlets using only straighteners, but there is a knack to the technique, and good tuition is essential if you want to avoid creating unsightly kinks in your hair. Luckily, beauty vlogger Riannstar, otherwise known as college student Riann, has created an easy-to-follow masterclass just for you. This is a great technique to use on long hair, and a skill that everyone should master, as it will open up a whole variety of looks for you using just one tool, which perhaps explains why this clever clip has been viewed more than 2.5 million times!

http://youtu.be/ArvvCtSj2us

Curl Hair with Straighteners: Shoulder-Length Hair

Kandee Johnson's curls tutorial for shorter locks

Mother-of-four Kandee Johnson is a highly successful makeup artist and vlogger. She manages to infuse her fun beauty tutorials with heaps of personality and humour, making her super-easy to watch. Here Kandee shows how you can create "crazy curls" on shoulder-length hair with a pair of hair straighteners: "the only hair tool you'll ever need". The cool Californian shows how wrapping hair in and around the irons and then slowing pulling it down creates big, perfectly rounded ringlets. The trick is to work section by section and keep your technique the same the whole way around your head. To finish the look, Kandee backcombs the roots, tousles everything with her fingers and rubs through a little oil to reduce frizz.

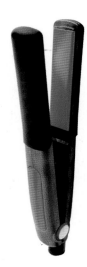

Big Hair Tutorial

Heated rollers made easy
with Dizzy Brunette

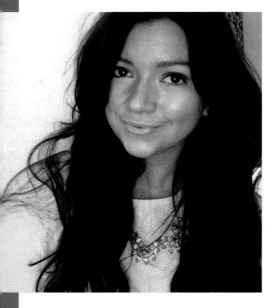

Corrie, aka DizzyBrunette3, is a UK beauty blogger who specializes in fabulous hair tutorials for long hair. Her presenting style is very approachable and tends to focus on affordable products, making her perfect for younger beauty addicts. Here she's enthusing about heated rollers, which can seem like way too much work, but Corrie makes it look easy. She starts by applying dry shampoo to add texture and lift to the roots of her hair, before demo-ing just how easy they are to put in, using the bigger size around the crown for added volume, and the smaller size on the underneath lengths. Twenty minutes later she whips them out and sprays over plenty of hairspray, before teasing everything into the shape she wants. Simple!

http://youtu.be/IZ-RRZRSCIc

Paper Bag Curls Tutorial

Michelle Phan's surprising method for heat-free curls

Since Michelle Phan began posting tutorials in 2007, she's gained more than 5 million followers to her eponymous channel and is now the most subscribed beauty guru on YouTube. This video is great because the "paper strip" method is simple and won't damage hair (as it doesn't require heat). Michelle makes it stylish too, using her favourite Hello Kitty paper bags, which she rips into vertical strips. She then wraps small sections of damp hair around the paper strips and twists – showing the technique up-close, so you quickly get the idea – before leaving her hair to dry overnight. In essence it's a modern take on old-fashioned rag rolling, but it sure does work, as Michelle unwraps a head of cascading curls the next day.

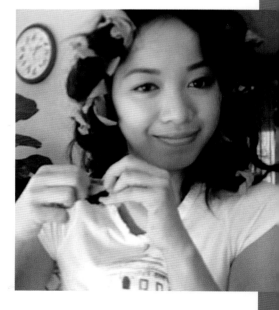

http://youtu.be/WoZ2QGq0n4A

Full Sexy Curls

Jessica Harlow hair-curling
tutorial

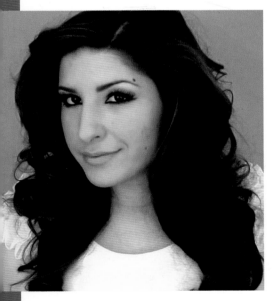

Jessica Harlow's upbeat and intimate manner makes
you feel like you're getting advice from a cool big
sister. Her videos are super-easy to follow but leave
you feeling ultra glamorous. Here she demos her
technique for perfect curls, which involves using
tongs on each section of hair and then taking the
curl they create and pinning it up on top of the head
with a bobby pin. She leaves everything to set for
15 minutes, then removes the pins, backcombs a
little and adds hairspray before she's good to go,
looking salon perfect. Her top tong tip is to always
use a heat defence spray to protect your hair.

http://youtu.be/6Nf4aZq4zhI

Wavy Curls for Spring

Put a spring in your hair
with MissGlamorazzi

There's nothing better than giving your hairstyling routine a spring clean by getting to grips with a fresh new look. Soft, bouncy, wavy curls topped off with a pretty hairband works well on brighter spring days and Ingrid Nilsen, aka YouTube megastar MissGlamorazzi, is here to demonstrate how she creates this romantic style. It couldn't be easier to achieve, as the Thai-Norwegian beauty walks you through every step from adding volume with a simple blow-dry technique, creating bouncy laid back curls and completing the look by making your own GIY (that's "glamorize it yourself") hairbands.

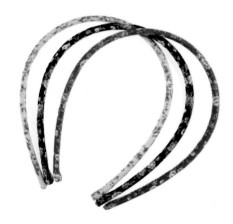

Clip Curl Technique

Luxy Hair's trick for curling
without damaging hair

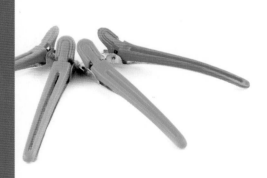

Sisters Mimi and Leyla are the founders of Luxy Hair, a hair extensions company, and have built a fantastic YouTube channel that's a must-see for anyone who loves experimenting with their hair. Heat damage from repeated use of curling tongs leads to split ends and can leave your hair feeling weak and brittle. But that's just the price you have to pay for bouncy curls, right? Well, not any more, as Mimi from Luxy Hair has invented this clever way to create cute curls without using any heat at all! All you need is hairspray, a spray bottle full of water, plenty of hair clips and your middle finger!

http://youtu.be/Vxws6YOOpmg

Set Naturally Curly Hair into Softer Waves

Learn to love your hair
with Hair Romance

Christina Butcher, the self-described "hair behind YouTube channel Hair Romance", used to hate her curly hair, but over time she's learnt to love her natural curls. In this, the first vlog she ever recorded, Christina demonstrates a softer wavy style that is incredibly easy to achieve. "I'm not a hairdresser," she says, "and I don't have any special training, so if I can do it, I know you can too." The look takes just 2 minutes to create and involves simply twisting up and pinning hair into little messy balls on top of your head while it's wet – you don't even need to look in a mirror while you do it, as Christina shows. When dry, the hair is simply unpinned and frizzy locks are magically replaced with softly tousled waves.

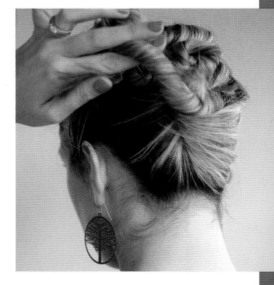

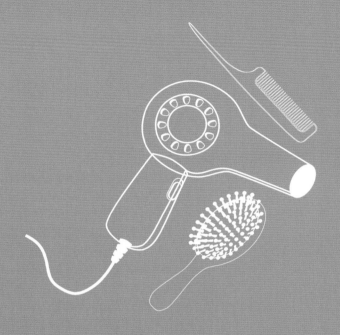

BLOWDRIES

and Styling Techniques

Easy Blowdry

Master the art of hairdrying
with Lo Bosworth

Lo Bosworth may have only been vlogging for a short time, but the former *Laguna Beach* and *The Hills* star has quickly built up an impressive following to her eponymous channel. Her tutorials often reveal clever beauty shortcuts or money-saving tricks to looking great, such as this blowdry guide. "It's pretty easy honestly," says Lo. "Just start with damp hair, a great dryer and a round brush – along with a bit of patience." Lo demos her own favourite technique for drying underneath first, followed by the top sections. She also shares a great tip of blowing against the direction in which you want the hair to fall for maximum volume.

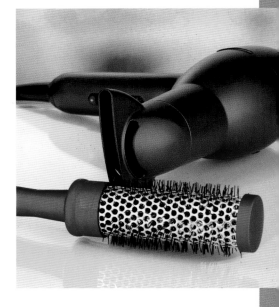

Which Styling Products and Tools *Really* Work?

Lisa Eldridge's inside track
on hair essentials

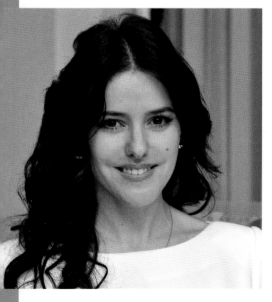

Lisa Eldridge is a highly experienced, London-based makeup artist who has worked with celebrities such as Kate Winslet and Keira Knightley. Her glossy, professional tutorials are packed with insider secrets. Here Lisa shares her favourite all-time hair products, including Kerastase volumizing shampoos and Wam hairdryers. She's also a big fan of leave-in hair creams and treatments, especially those containing the latest wonder ingredient, argan oil, which helps boost hair hydration. However, she warns against using these products at the roots or they will weigh down hair. When it comes to curl creation, however, the professional stylist favours cheap, basic curling tongs or old-school heated rollers.

http://youtu.be/Gn9DJWsideQ

How to Style Curly Hair

Let your hair's natural beauty shine through with AndreasChoice

With advice on everything beauty-related, plus a knack for not taking herself too seriously on camera, American vlogger Andrea Brooks has attracted 2.5 million subscribers to her channel AndreasChoice. This video explains Andrea's own routine for styling her gorgeous, naturally curly locks, with no products required. She starts by simply combing through with a wide-tooth comb, but her most important tip is to re-wet hair with water spray and scrunch it – as this encourages the strands to curl up and stick together. Next she shows us how to use a diffuser hairdryer attachment, which we're told takes longer than a normal dryer, but gives by far the best results on curls.

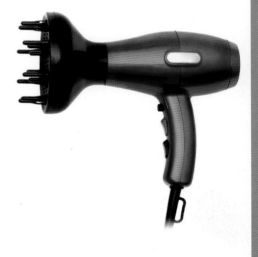

Blowdry Your Hair – No Sweat

Michelle Phan shares her
professional hair secrets

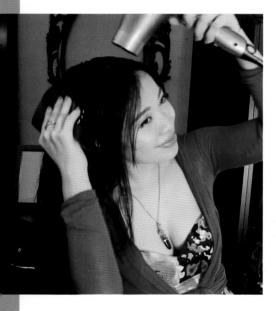

In this video that has racked up more than 2.5 million views, Boston blogger Michelle Phan gives her take on blowdrying. Start with a lightweight PH-based shampoo and conditioner and then apply a heat-protecting spray, before drying hair 80–90 per cent dry on a warm to cool setting. If it gets too hot, Michelle warns that the outer hair surface will dry out while the inner hair core remains moist, causing "steam blisters" which will make it look dull, dry and even break off – yikes! A big fan of the round brush, Michelle's other insider tip is to get a hairdryer with an A/C motor – favoured by most hair professionals – rather than the less effective D/C motor found in the majority of consumer dryers.

http://youtu.be/N6w4fH-3RiA

A "Big Hair" Party Look

Add volume to shoulder-length locks with Pixiwoo

Samantha and Nic Chapman are the makeup artist sisters behind one of the best-known beauty vlogs – Pixiwoo. Here Sam shows how heated rollers can be used to create a "big hair" party look. Invaluable technique tips include making sure the ends of your hair are tucked in when you roll to avoid crinkling, and getting the roller as close to the roots as possible for maximum volume. Sam also rolls away from the parting, maintaining tension while rolling for an even curl, and sprays with hairspray once they're in. Just 15 minutes later, when the rollers have cooled down, Sam shows how to take them out and separate the hair, adding a tiny amount of texture powder at the roots for a final bit of oomph.

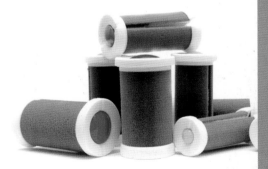

Perfectly Tousled Tresses

 Master the lived-in look
with I Covet Thee

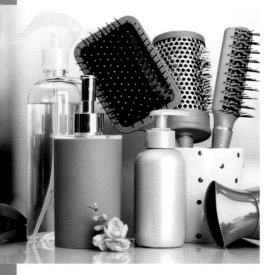

Alix from I Covet Thee's true forte lies in creating simple tutorials, outlining gorgeous everyday hair and beauty routines. Watch here as the Brit blogger and vlogger shows every step of her hairstyling routine, from the products she applies to how she dries her fringe (bangs) first, and works hard to get extra volume into the side and back sections. In her words: "I'm a fan of the 'just rolled out of bed with perfectly tousled hair' look, although for me it takes hours of messing around and applying products to achieve!" The graphic-led video is dialogue-free with a infectiously chirpy soundtrack. This quirky approach allows you to concentrate on the technical aspects of her look.

http://youtu.be/8Ul7cdYwU6c

Bohemian Summer Hair

Get the festival look with MakeupByAlli

Makeup-obsessed Alli shows viewers how to keep their beauty fresh and fun, and her tutorials are perfect for those who love natural-looking hairstyles. The bohemian look she covers in this clip is the perfect style for a weekend festival, says Alli, because it's low maintenance and will last for up to three days. She begins by blowdrying her hair until 90 per cent dry, and then applies styling mousse all over. She then proceeds to twist her hair in small sections, from top to bottom, before using the diffuser on it and scrunching. Next there's some light "tonging", before Alli adds some texture spray and then "fluffs it up" to create a last bit of volume.

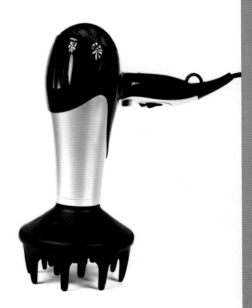

"I Just Had Sex" Hair Tutorial

Jessica Harlow brings out
your inner siren

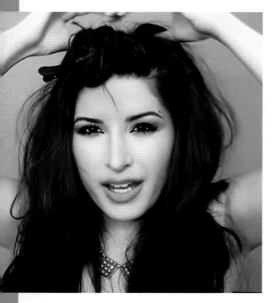

Sophia Loren once said: "Sex appeal is fifty per cent what you've got, and fifty per cent what people think you've got." So if you want to exude steamy sex appeal, then follow this advice from US vlogger Jessica Harlow on how to fake that "just-got-out-of-bed-after-y'know" soft, tousled look. Jessica has lovely full hair, but she has plenty of advice on faking thickness if you're not so naturally blessed, including how to create "air pockets" that will make your hair appear fuller. Don't miss her backcombing technique that won't damage your hair, and her "flip and shake" technique to revive the look throughout the day.

http://youtu.be/4UAm-p36exU

Temporary Dreadlocks Hair Tutorial

Emma Pickles goes for grunge

Yorkshire-based beauty blogger Emma Pickles creates some of the most innovative and exciting beauty tutorials on YouTube, and this look is no exception as we're shown how to rock some authentic-looking dreadlocks. She demos her twist, braid and backcomb technique for creating dreads, starting with the bottom section of her hair. She then rubs and sprays hairspray over each piece to hold it in place. The end look is very effective, and while not for everyone, would be perfect for a 1980s-themed party, as it has more than a hint of Boy George back in his Culture Club days about it.

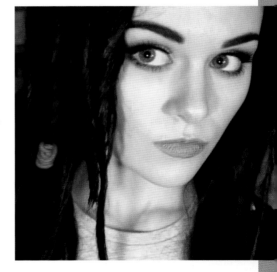

http://youtu.be/zIIw5H0KtYs

How to Style Your Fringe

Get through the awkward in-between stage with Essie Button

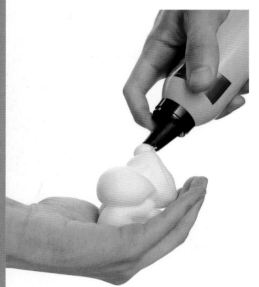

If you have fine hair, Estée, aka Essie Button, should be your go-to vlogger for product recommendations and tips. And if you're in the painful process of growing out your fringe (bangs), or looking for advice on how to style a longer fringe, this video is an absolute must see. Estée's fringe is at that awkward in-between stage where it's too long to be a proper fringe but too short to blend back in with the rest of her hair. Thankfully, the England-based Canadian has found a simple way to keep it looking sleek and polished while it grows out. Her techniques are guaranteed to keep the front of your hair looking bouncy and fresh, however long it is.

http://youtu.be/FO8wPzKYcKc

Post-Gym Hair SOS

Tanya Burr's tips on fixing
your hair after a workout

Even tied back in a ponytail, a hard gym workout
can leave hair looking sweaty, limp and lifeless.
Thankfully beauty vlogger extraordinaire, Tanya Burr,
has created this masterclass on how to breathe life
back into your locks, so they're full of movement –
perfect for when you don't have time to wash it
properly before heading to your next appointment.
Her secret method is to run a good spritz of dry
shampoo all over to absorb grease and add some
bounce. The English vlogger's other fab trick is then
to blast your hair with a hairdryer, which cleverly
creates as much volume as if you've actually washed
and blowdried it from scratch!

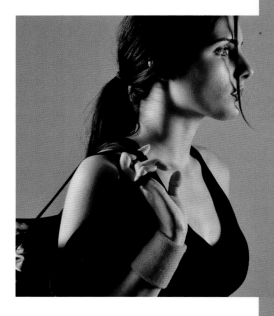

http://youtu.be/MR7-3a4kFps

Get Your Best "Twist Out" Ever

Naptural85's stretched-out
twist masterclass

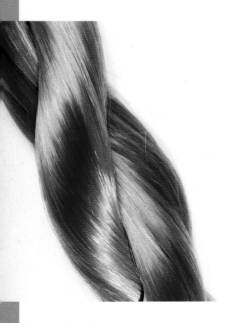

For those not in the know, a "twist out" is a hairdo, usually done on naturally curly hair, where you two-strand twist the hair when wet and allow it to dry, before untwisting to style. Natural hair guru Whitney, aka Naptural85, is here to show you how to improve your twist-out technique so that you achieve the best results every time. The key is to start by getting rid of your natural curl pattern, so that your hair can adapt to the zigzag curl pattern of your twist, which means before twisting it must first be straightened. But wait… isn't Whitney famed for not using damaging heat on her hair? Fear not, the vlogger knows a top tip for faking that straighter shape, as well as how to define and elongate twists to the max.

http://youtu.be/ruRGEe3DfOY

How to Add Hair "Oomph"

I Covet Thee's tips for creating fuller-looking hair

Alix of I Covet Thee describes her natural hair as flat, limp and fine, but you'd never know that, as she's mastered a technique for adding volume to hair to create the illusion of a thick, bouncy mane. Here she demonstrates how she uses a curling wand and hairspray to create a style she favours when she wants something quick and easy, but with a lot of voluminous curls. Learn why it's important not to twist hair as you wind it around a curling iron and how to brush hair up, rather than down, to create a tousled look that will last all day.

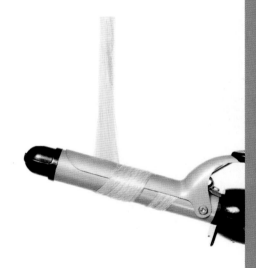

Chic Faux Bob

Fake a dramatic chop
with Annie Jaffrey

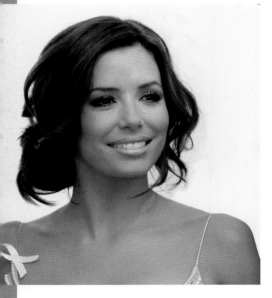

This chic look was inspired by the idea of #ThrowBackThursday, a popular social media meme which has seen celebrities and fashionistas posting old photos of themselves every Thursday. The idea of turning back the clock prompted vlogger Annie Jaffrey to create this vintage look. Learn how to quickly transform long locks into a cute 1950s-style retro bob without actually cutting off any of your hair. As Annie says, this simple technique "totally changes up your look within minutes, without making any permanent decisions." Turn up to a party with this cropped style and prepare to draw a few shocked gasps from friends and family members!

http://youtu.be/v03yNCXPq0s

The Faux Side Shave

Try an edgier look
with StillGlamorus

Rihanna, Kelly Osborne and even young Willow Smith have rocked the edgy side-shaved style, which was first popularized in the late 1980s and early '90s by the likes of rap duo Salt-N-Pepa. It's a dramatic look, but if you're not brave enough to go for the close shave, you'll be pleased to learn that, with the help of this informative vlog from StillGlamorus, it's a relatively easy look to fake. And it turns out there's no shame in favouring the faux style over the real one, as the Arizonan vlogger (real name Kasey Marie Palmer) reveals Beyoncé, Jessica Alba, Kristen Stewart and Ke$ha have all faked it.

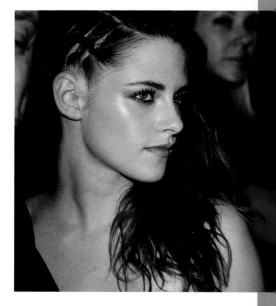

http://youtu.be/dvnLZBwAlZY

Add Volume to Straight, Fine Hair

Get fuller locks with Essie Button

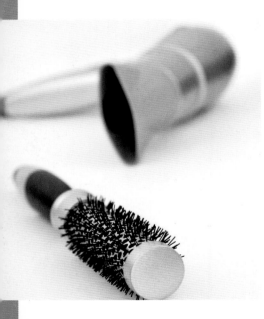

Do you normally discount volume-boosting tutorials because they tend to rely on your hair having a certain level of thickness and volume to begin with? If you thought your thin hair was beyond saving and that "bounce" was something for other people, then this is the vlog for you. Essie knows your pain – her hair is ultra fine, but she has found the best products and styling techniques to give it extra oomph. This is a realistic tutorial that doesn't claim to be able to help you create big Beyoncé hair, but does make a striking difference to limp locks.

http://youtu.be/8iJ-vW1Vg9U

The Lazy Girl's Guide to Everyday Hair

Elle Fowler's minimum fuss, maximum style routine

Let's be honest, we all have days when we're tired, fed up or just plain can't be bothered to spend hours styling our hair. Thankfully, YouTube celebrity Elle Fowler knows a simple and fast way to get hair looking good with the minimum fuss and effort required. Here she outlines how applying a leave-in serum to wet hair will make it look instantly smoother and shinier when dry. Not one for sectioning off hair and fiddling with brushes, once it's had a quick blast with the hairdryer, Elle's top tip is to run through your entire mop quickly with straighteners to banish any frizz – then she's all primped and ready to go.

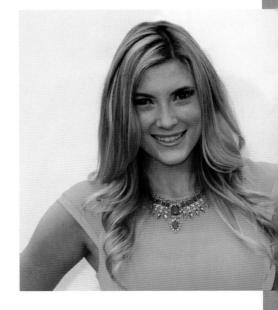

http://youtu.be/2dgpp_hQZYY

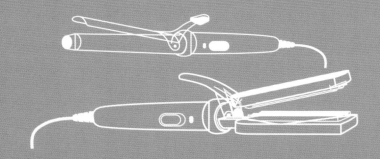

STRAIGHTENING

and Hair Extensions

Stress-Free Straightening

Bethany Mota's straightening session for beginners

Millions of young girls are familiar with young beauty vlogger Bethany Mota, who has built herself a media and fashion empire – all from the comfort of her Californian bedroom. And it's not hard to see why, with her easy delivery style and enthusiasm. Here she tells us how much she loves her GHD straighteners and why she uses a heat protector spray to ensure they don't fry her hair. She also confesses that she can't be bothered to section her locks before styling, so she just goes from one side to the next with the straightener until it's all sleek, which she finds works just as well, if not even better.

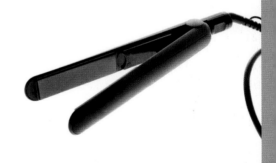

http://youtu.be/4uDK5t0Hf9Y

How to Straighten Curly Hair

Go straight with
Cassandra Bankson

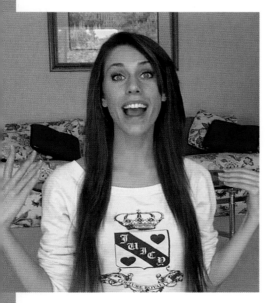

Cassandra Bankson is a model and self-employed beauty guru who boasts a huge archive of videos on her channel DiamondsAndHeels14, including this popular clip detailing how she straightens her curly hair. Great tips include using the concentrator nozzle and cool button on your dryer, as they will help flatten the hair cuticle for added shine, plus prevent hair becoming too frazzled. Cassandra works methodically with the straighteners, going in sections from back to front, and advises that with very curly hair, the smaller the piece you take each time and the slower you go, the better it works. The end result? Super-shiny, sleek locks.

http://youtu.be/Xms2pZjG44w

No Heat Tutorial for Straight Hair

DelanySmiles' secret to straightening without an iron

Delaney has discovered the holy grail of healthy hairstyling: how to achieve poker-straight hair without using damaging heated tools. She's not the most prolific of vloggers and her YouTube channel has just 14,000 subscribers, but this video has racked up more than a million views, as this is one technique that you have to see to believe. Delaney promises that this heat-free technique – involving a household fan – can straighten naturally curly hair without damaging it. She also helpfully points out that, contrary to what you may have heard, cool air and wet hair won't give you a cold!

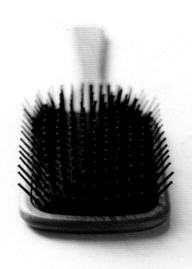

How to Use Clip-in Hair Extensions

Fake long shiny locks in seconds with Ruth Crilly

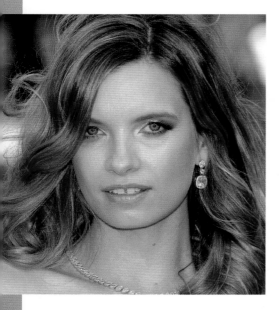

British model Ruth Crilly is founder of one of the world's best-known beauty blogs, A Model Recommends. Her YouTube makeup tutorials use insider secrets to create fabulous results but are all explained in a clear, easy-to-follow manner. Here she shows how to use clip-in hair extensions to add loads of volume and length, without the hassle and expense of going to a salon to have them fitted – or the bother of growing your own hair long! Her top tips for ensuring extensions don't fall out include not using them on freshly washed hair and applying some "backcomb dust" – a styling powder that gives hair extra texture and grip.

http://youtu.be/K0PA_LCkVn8

Fake Big, Sexy Hair

Sona Gasparian's guide to curly extensions

LA-based professional makeup artist Sona Gasparian runs the popular YouTube channel MakeupBySona, which is packed with fun hair tutorials. In this guide to using real hair clip-in extensions she demos how to curl them with tongs first, repeating the tong technique on her own hair so the two match. Then she simply clips the extensions in at the sides and back, hiding the join lines under her own hair. The result is messy '70s-style curls, with extra length and volume for a seriously sexy look. Perfect for a special night out – and you can simply unclip and take the extensions out when you get back home!

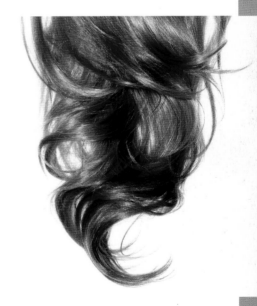

http://youtu.be/iCwyPT7VkZQ

Make Your Own Clip-On Fringe

Get instant bangs
with Michelle Phan

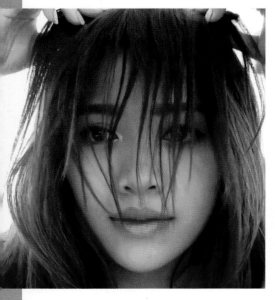

Michelle Phan's YouTube tutorials average several million views, and this nifty clip has likewise proved pretty popular, despite its less obvious subject matter. The video details how to make yourself a fake fringe (bangs), using some long clip-in hair extensions bought from the local pharmacy, colour-matched to your own hair shade. Watch as Michelle lays the hair over her face to work out the correct length before cutting the extensions to fit. Her top trick is to use two layers of slightly different shades for a more natural look. When your fringe is ready, Michelle shows you how to clip it seamlessly into your own hair. Perfect for trying a fringe without the long-term commitment.

http://youtu.be/YHRZ7mV20v0

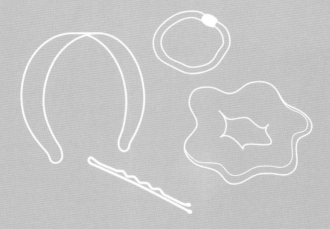

PLAITS

and Ponies

Volumized Ponytail

Jessica Harlow takes ponytails
out of high school

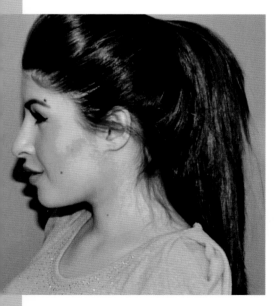

Vlogger Jessica Harlow likes to focus on timeless hair trends, as opposed to throw-away fashion looks. Here she creates a classic ponytail that's grown-up and sophisticated, making it perfect for a prom or ball. She begins by straightening her hair to ensure it is sleek and glossy, and explains it's worth running the irons over your hair, even if it's naturally straight, because getting it super-smooth before putting it up will make the finished style look far more polished. Watch out for her clever trick of hiding the hair band with a strand of her own hair. Simple, but oh so stylish.

http://youtu.be/IdWd_egmWvA

Cute Heart-Shaped Braids

Fall in love with
Bubzbeauty plaits

You can't help but warm to perky Irish vlogger Lindy
Tsang of Bubzbeauty, so it's no wonder her cute,
easy-to-follow hair and makeup tutorials have
attracted 2.7 million subscribers. This is a pretty
hairstyle that is great for everyday, as Lindy explains:
"I usually do it whenever I have bad hair days. It
works because it looks great messy or neat and the
braid is unique because it looks like little hearts."
You start simply with two normal-size plaits (braids)
and then the magic begins as Lindy pulls out little
sections of the plait so they sit away from the main
plait. The end result? A really cool, unusual shape
that will draw compliments wherever you go.

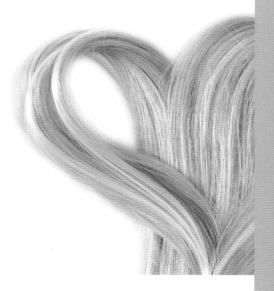

http://youtu.be/pGfqlkZQkQ8?list

Braided Waves

Boho chic with
Bethany Mota

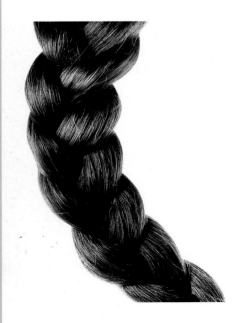

Bethany Mota is one of the top three biggest YouTube beauty celebrities, with nearly 5 million subscribers to her channel. Her style is fun but she's not short of helpful how-tos either. The mixture of curls and plaits (braids) Bethany creates in this popular clip is her favourite spring hairstyle. She starts by taking a hair section at the front and on the side, and braiding it tightly to the scalp until you reach the ear. She then uses a cone-shaped curling tong to create some soft curls in the unbraided hair, finishes everything with a little hairspray, and *voilà*! – it's done – all in less than 5 minutes. A great holiday look.

http://youtu.be/VIgT2pWo1qM

The Five-Strand Braid

Create the ultimate plait
with Luxy Hair

Known for their beautiful step-by-step hair tutorials, Luxy Hair make styling look simple. Here, Luxy's Mimi demonstrates the ultimate in plaiting (braiding) – the five-strand braid. Thankfully, as this video shows us, this ambitious look is actually easier to create than you might think, and is a perfect daytime hairstyle for work or school. The secret to nailing the look is "invisible" transparent hair bands to hold everything in place. Mimi also recommends repeating the mantra of "Over… Under" to ensure you remember which way to braid each strand. The end results are stunning – like shiny, woven silk. A skill well worth mastering.

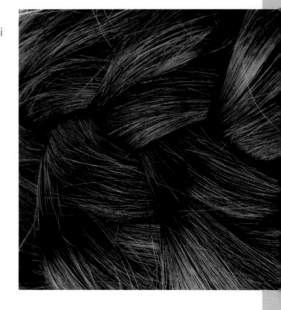

Thicker-Looking Hair Braid

Fake high-volume hair
with MissChievous

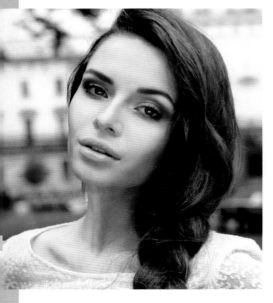

Julia Graf creates incredible hair and makeup vlogs on her MissChievous YouTube channel, which no beauty lover should miss. Here she reveals that because her own hair is very fine, she's constantly trying to come up with ways to make it look thicker, as with this funky side braid. Her secret is to add plenty of volume before plaiting (braiding), using both styling powder and texture spray, and a teensy bit of backcombing. This look is fab in itself, but Julia also demos a clever way to transform it into an updo by pinning the braid on top of your head for evening chic.

http://youtu.be/pxYGlHEBY1o

Scallop Braid Headband

Make waves with Bebexo's mermaid-style hair

From formal updos to intricate braids, Bebexo vlogger Nee promises creative tutorials for all hair lengths. This half-up do works on medium or longer hair and involves braiding the front and side sections, using an amazing technique of dropping a piece of hair to create a striking "scallop" effect. It sounds complicated, but thankfully Nee shows it's simple if you take it slowly. Both plaits (braids) then meet at the back and are tied together. The end result is a gorgeous sculpted shape that's special enough for a night out but still casual enough to wear in the day.

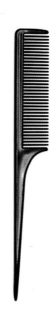

Soft Dutch Braid

Abby Smith twists
herself pretty

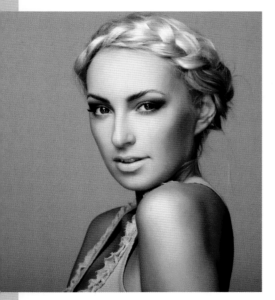

Abby Smith, a stay-at-home mother of two, initially began beauty vlogging as a way of pulling together all the style looks she loved. Before long her collection became Twist Me Pretty, a YouTube channel where you'll find a myriad of incredible hairstyles for every occasion. To show just how to create this attractive Dutch braid, Abby makes clever use of slow motion so you don't miss a step. Watch carefully, as this is one of those fiddly multi-strand styles. Her top tip is not to look in the mirror as you do it, or you'll become confused! Also watch out for her braid-pulling technique to add volume at the end. Hard work but well worth it.

http://youtu.be/G7v-ny5Nkgk

A Ponytail for All Occasions

Evening hair glamour with
Emily Noel Eddington

Emily Eddington started her career as a US news anchor before leaving to run her hugely successful YouTube beauty channel, emilynoel83, full-time. And her experience really shines through in her clear and confident delivery style. Here she shows how a few simple tricks can make a ponytail suitable for a glam night out. Her top tip is to section off and backcomb the front section, securing it with a hairgrip, rather than pulling it up into the main pony. She also demonstrates a clever way to make an "x" shape with the two grips to ensure they stay put all night.

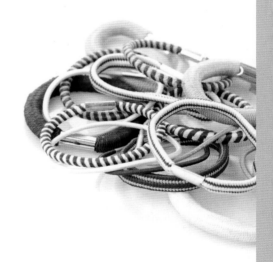

How to Create a Waterfall Plait

Tanya Burr's perfect
hippy braid

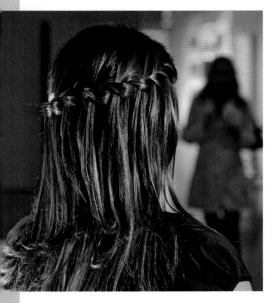

Brilliant Brit Tanya Burr is one of the most watched beauty vloggers and has trained with professionals all over the world. Tanya believes great hair styling is all about the prep, so washing and conditioning your locks the night before is vital, ideally with texturising products so they're not too slippery. This casual braid is a trendy Boho look, so she just plaits (braids) one side, loosely and not too neatly. It take less than 3 minutes to do, which means it would be a perfect festival look – especially for second- or third-day festival hair as it will neatly hide the fact it's been a while since its last proper wash.

http://youtu.be/_tVtjjfTH7s

Diagonal French Loop Braid

One for the girls with Mindy McKnight

As a mother to five girls herself, Utah-based Mindy McKnight, creator of Cute Girls Hairstyles channel, certainly knows a thing or two about making girls' hair look pretty. She starting vlogging to give other mums ideas for their daughters' hair, and often uses her own girls as models for her tutorials. This incredibly striking plait (braid) is a real show-stopper and would be perfect for an end-of-year school party or show. Mindy's top – and rather unusual – tip is to braid while hair is wet; apparently this makes the process easier and neater. You'll need a willing participant with an extra pair of hands to hold sections for this one.

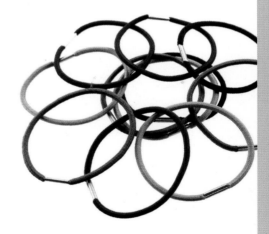

http://youtu.be/BWO_MUiVchQ

Fake a Longer, Thicker Ponytail

Naptural85's nifty trick for making hair look fuller

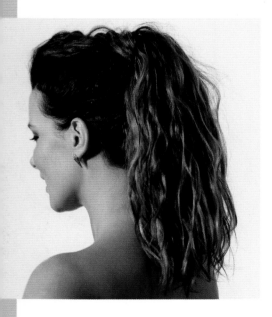

Ponytails look great when they are thick and full, but they have the potential to come across as lacklustre and humdrum if your hair is lacking in body and length. So what can you do on days when your hair is looking a little limp? Let Whitney, aka Naptural85, show you her simple trick for making your hair look twice as full and thrice as long in 3 minutes flat. Watch as she divides hair into two ponytails, which she then cleverly disguises as one thick bunch that reaches from the top of the head to the nape of the neck.

http://youtu.be/m1N7H61ffuc

Twisted Fishtail Braid Tutorial

Fleur DeForce's fabulous fishy technique

Northampton girl Fleur is the self-styled "makeup obsessive" behind beauty fashion and lifestyle YouTube channel, FleurDeForce. She's attracted more than a million dedicated followers with her friendly girl-next-door manner and sage beauty advice. In this vlog she demonstrates how to create a messy and romantic twisted fishtail plait (braid). This is a great look for windy winter days, as it will stop your hair getting knotted, and using Fleur's method it is super-easy to achieve. Don't miss her tips for adding volume or her guide to creating either a chunky, funky fishtail or a delicate detailed one.

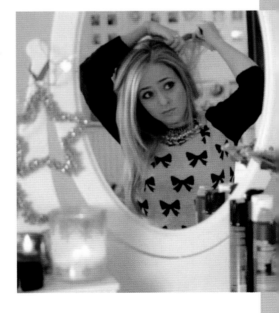

http://youtu.be/BU3mdp-oe3c

Messy Faux Fishtail Side Braid Tutorial

Lo Bosworth's trick for faking
a professional finish

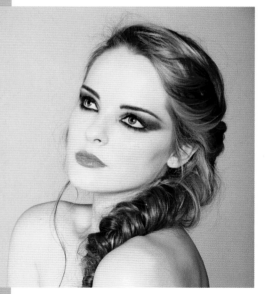

Fishtail plaits (braids) are a statement look. More textured and intricate than run-of-the-mill plaits, they are guaranteed to draw envious glances from women who have tried, but failed, to master the technique themselves. Unsurprisingly, it is a tricky look, which often requires two pairs of hands and a bit of time. But Lo Bosworth has invented a simple twisting technique, which creates the appearance of a fishtail plait but in less than half the time. The technique requires far less fiddly sectioning, so it's also easy to achieve on your own. (We won't tell anyone it's not a real fishtail braid, if you won't!)

http://youtu.be/PwqGwvMsVZc

High Ponytail with Curls

Blair Fowler's tips for
adding glamour

One day Blair Fowler decided to go to a party with
her hair in a high pony simply because she didn't
have time to wash it. Next morning the Juicystar07
vlogger awoke to a twitterfeed full of requests for
a tutorial showing how she created the "statement
updo". Of course the look is actually super simple
and quick to recreate once you know Blair's little
tricks and tips. In this clip the younger Fowler sister
shows how to ensure your pony is bouncy, using
tongs to create spiral curls and securing it in position
at the "tippy top" of your head, and how to ensure it
keeps its volume throughout the night.

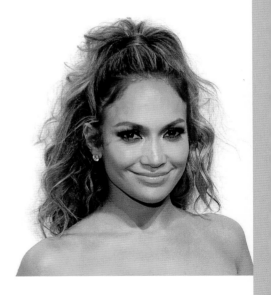

Triple Twisted Ponytail

Twist Me Pretty's "fun twist"
on a traditional pony

This look from Twist Me Pretty's resident blonde Abby Smith is a fun twist (pardon the pun) on the traditional ponytail. The style requires twisting sections of hair before securing it up in a pony, adding a romantic edge and making it reminiscent of the flowing hair of a Disney princess. A fitting comparison when you learn that as well as vlogging, the all-American working mom is also a beauty writer for Disney. Abby's helpful hints: If you have flyaway hair, make sure you use a good hairspray, and if you feel like the hairpins aren't holding things in place enough, double them up.

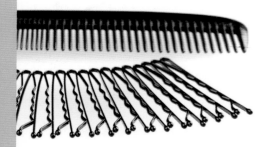

http://youtu.be/U3REMItznz8?list

Milkmaid Braid

Pretty plaiting technique from
The Beauty Department

Learn how to create this traditional look with help
from The Beauty Department's resident hair guru
Kristin Ess. This popular YouTube channel was
launched by US reality TV star Lauren Conrad, her
makeup artist, Amy Nadine, and her hairstylist,
Kristin, with the aim of teaching beauty basics and
trends. In this vlog Kristin shows you how easy it is
create this lovely updo, which involves two side
plaits (braids) that meet on top of the head. Watch
out for the great tips on making the look your own
by weaving a thin fabric through the braids, and how
to soften the finish by using a crochet hook to pull
hair a little looser. Any version is a great look for
summer festivals.

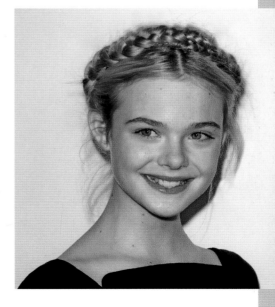

Perfect Ponytail with Ruth Crilly

A "bad hair day" remedy
from All Things Hair

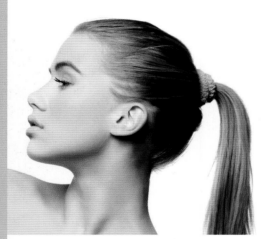

Ponytails: they look so simple, but they can often turn out to be a right pain in the (back of the) neck. Trying to get a classic, smooth, bump-free style, which isn't too tight or too loose, can drive you to the point of pulling your hair out. Ruth Crilly, the vlogger behind A Model Recommends, has teamed up with YouTube channel All Things Hair to bring you this step-by-step guide to creating a ponytail that is not too flat or too poofy, but just right. Once you have mastered this look you can guarantee a happy ending to every ponytail.

http://youtu.be/lzQ4z2H7zDE

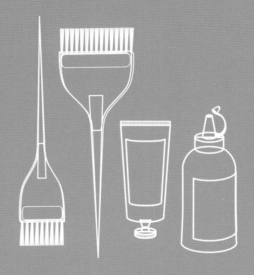

DYEING

Techniques

How to Honey-Dip Hair

Save money at the hairdresser
with Patricia Bright's DIY dye job

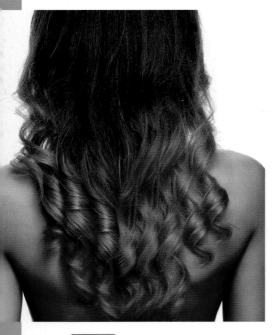

London-based blogger Patricia Bright talks you through this look – a cross between highlights and ombre (aka dip-dye) hair – which she calls "honey-dipping". The technique involves lightening the hair tips halfway to the root in a warmer, lighter shade. Patricia does all this from the comfort of her own home, using a simple pharmacy-bought highlighting kit – "it's really easy to do", she assures us. And in this 5-minute clip on the BritPopPrincess channel she shows us how mix the colour and – wearing gloves and old clothes – apply to the hair tips before leaving for 30 minutes. Once dry, the colour change is pretty impressive and you'll soon be itching for a dipping of your own.

http://youtu.be/kuRzz4orjYM

Get Pastel Lilac Hair

Create a purple hair haze
with Hannah Leigh

Hannah Leigh is a beauty blogger with a speciality in interesting and highly original DIY videos. She can teach you anything from how to make your own lipstick, to how to dip-dye your own hair. Here she walks us though how to get light purple hair. The first step, she explains, is to dye your hair a bleach blonde shade. Once lightened, to counteract those brassy yellow tones, Hannah recommends using a silvery hair toner, which won't further damage hair and so can be left on for a long time to ensure you get the right shade. Then it's time for the lilac, which she uses to bold effect. Finally she advises investing in a purple shampoo to maintain the colour.

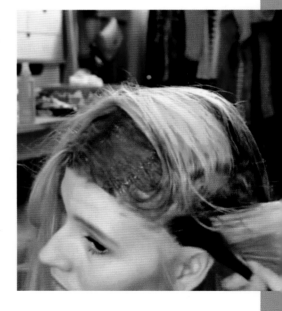

Golden Brown to Ash Brown Hair

Banish red from your tresses
with Weylie

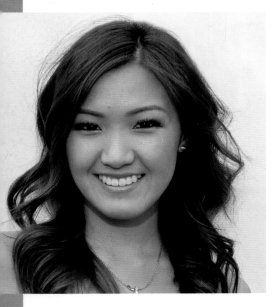

Trying to dye Asian or naturally dark hair a golden ash brown colour without bleaching it is tricky because, as Weylie, of ilikeweylie, says, "Our hair naturally has a really strong orange base." It's even trickier for Weylie, as her hair used to be dyed bright "Rihanna red", a look she wanted to ditch for an ash tone because "seriously girl, that is just not cute anymore, ok." Luckily, Weylie's discovered exactly the right type of dye for cancelling out red tones. The Chinese-American is a chatty girl and that's half the fun of her vlogs, but if you'd rather get straight to the tutorial, skip to 5:50 minutes.

http://youtu.be/rIMp9Fkzq-M

How to Go Properly Pink

Melon Lady gets hair inspiration from the toy pony world

Helen Anderson, aka Melon Lady, is a vlogger for lovers of a more alternative, daring beauty look. She's outrageous, outgoing and fun, but has attracted nearly 300,000 subscribers by offering lots of useful hair and makeup tutorials, including top ones on styling and caring for bleached hair. Here, in one of her most watched videos – which she dubs her "My Little Pony Hair Experiment" – Helen mixes a variety of dye colours to achieve a shocking pink effect. Even if the pony look is too OTT for you, it's a useful tutorial for anyone afraid of hair dye as Helen chucks the stuff on with no fear, although you might prefer to wear gloves after seeing the colour of her hands by the end!

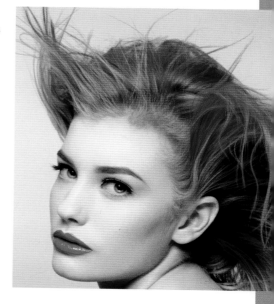

http://youtu.be/dQtU7141CBA

How to Dye Your Hair

The funny girl's guide to home-dyeing with Grace Helbig

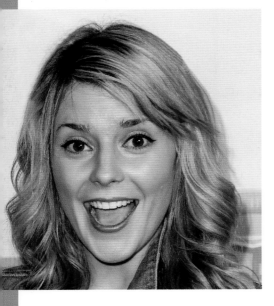

Grace Helbig, aka "Daily Grace", is one of vlogging's comedic gems, and now she's branching out into beauty how-tos. Which means you really must watch this clip because it's every bit as funny as it is helpful. Grace is quick to point out that home dyeing can be trial and error and it's foolish to expect hair exactly like the model on the packet of dye. This clip is in fact Grace's third attempt – thankfully all the swearing is bleeped out! Although you might not learn any professional hair secrets here, the 28-year-old American does show you how easy it is to change your hair colour at home – and her final results are in fact very much like the picture on the box.

http://youtu.be/hEx9RcRil8M

Ombre Pink and Purple Hair

Destiny Godley shows how to jazz up a blonde wig

Gorgeous vlogger Destiny Godley is an expert in black skin and hair techniques and is here to teach you everything from how to do your makeup like Rihanna, to natural ways to style your hair. Here she shows how to take a blonde wig and dye it purple with pink ombre tips – with impressive results. Destiny expertly mixes her dye, sharing tips on how to ensure an even colour when using such vibrant shades, and how to layer the two colours using foil. The eye-catching end product would be perfect for a special party, and best of all, because it's only a hair piece, you don't have to worry about growing out the colour when you've had enough of it!

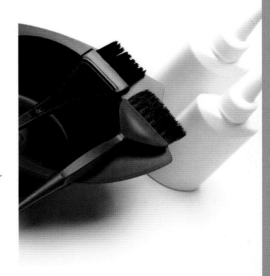

How to Colour Your Hair Salon-Style

The dye technique Kandee Johnson
learned at beauty school

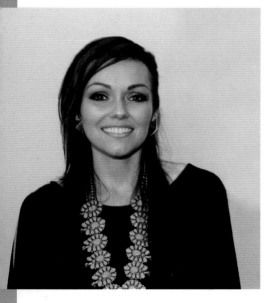

Kandee Johnson tells us her hair has been every colour under the sun, from bleach blonde to pitch black – not forgetting neon pink, traffic light green and Jessica Rabbit red! Turns out, makeup artist Kandee studied hair colouring at beauty school, so if you want to know about hair dye, she's your go-to gal. For anyone considering skipping the salon and dyeing your hair at home this clip is a must-watch with tips on how to avoid common mistakes such as missed patches, uneven colour and skin dyed the same colour as your hair. All told, with this tutorial you can get a professional-looking dye job at home for a fraction of the price.

http://youtu.be/fv2lo96heJU

DIY Hair Lightener

AndreasChoice lightens hair without a lemon in sight

Have you ever tried to lighten your hair in the sun using lemon juice? Then you'll know that rather than leaving you with the natural highlights you'd hoped for, this technique is more likely to result in frizzy, frazzled locks. But there is another kitchen ingredient that can naturally lighten hair without causing sun damage, and YouTube megastar Andrea Brooks of AndreasChoice is here to reveal that mystery hair hero. You'll never guess which kitchen cupboard staple is a natural source of peroxide! In fact Andrea demonstrates not one, but two ways to naturally lighten your hair without any professional assistance (or any lemons) but instead using a jar of honey.

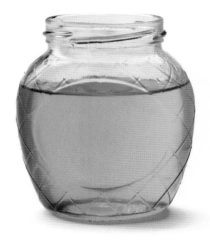

How to Dye Your Hair White, Silver or Grey

Helen Melon Lady's colour-stripping technique

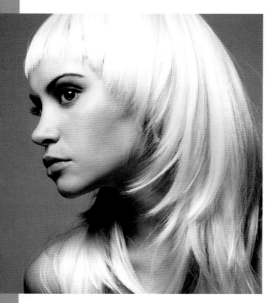

When you start watching this vlog you may think you've clicked on the wrong link, but don't worry, this isn't a 6-minute ode to Helen Melon Lady's pet Jetson: "the cutest dog in the world". Once the puppy love is over, the sparky Brit vlogger starts to explain exactly how you can strip all colour from your hair to make it white, silver or grey. Indispensable tips include how to avoid common bleaching problems, like hair that is lighter at the roots than on the ends. She also spills her secrets for maintaining the look and preventing your white hair from going brassy or green.

http://youtu.be/epy-B_CZHW8

How to Create Leopard-Print Hair

Brave this fierce style with
How-To Hair Girl

Are you a fan of leopard-print clothes? Why not take the statement print to a whole new level by sporting animal spots in your hair (celery is used to create the pattern)! Roxie Jane Hunt, the hairstylist behind this edgy vlog, wants to encourage women to ignore negative messages telling them they need to look a certain way to be "beautiful". Her inspirational videos are about finding a unique look that is "the gateway to your identity". So if your true personality is a fierce feline that will not change its spots, then this inspiring watch will certainly help you display your inner wild cat!

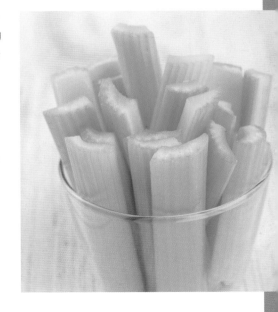

http://youtu.be/DpYYnYmDBEc

DIY Ombre Halo Highlights

Frame your face with highlights
like Kandee Johnson

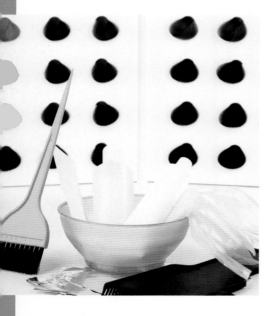

Ombre (otherwise known as dip-dye) styling is bang on-trend, with celeb fans including Lea Michele, Alexandra Burke and Jessica Biel. But why follow what everyone else is doing when, with a simple alteration, you can stand out from the crowd? For a more original take on this popular look, check out Kandee Johnson's technique for creating a halo effect around your face. "I wanted to frame my face with highlights instead of just making it look like the tips of my hair were dipped in bleach or like my roots had just grown out," the LA lifestyle blogger explains.

http://youtu.be/FPVsWpC0wps

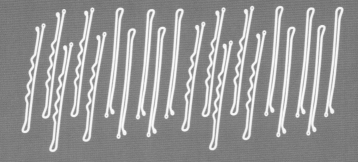

UPDOS

and Half-up Styles

Twisty Updo

Go for Grecian glamour
with Annie Jaffrey

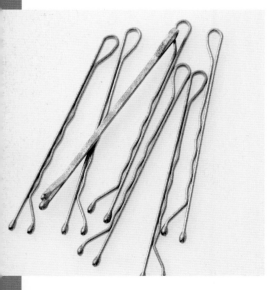

Beauty and health food guru Annie Jaffrey believes that healthy hair can be achieved only by a combination of eating a nutritious diet and using the right products – and if her silky locks are anything to go by, it's advice well worth heeding. In this updo tutorial she starts by liberally spritzing hair with dry shampoo to add some grip, before twisting her hair inwards, all the way around, securing it with hair pins as she goes. She then rolls up the remaining hair at the back, again pinning neatly. Watch out for her bun scrunching tips to give everything a lived-in, natural look and for the final addition of shine spray to get that perfect glossy finish.

http://youtu.be/hz-3-sY2FTM?list

Simple Romantic Updo

Channel some hair love with
Michelle Phan

If you're after a simple style that radiates romance, then look no further. This vlog from YouTube megastar Michelle Phan will teach you how to create an easy updo that is super soft and begging to be touched. For this clip, Michelle hands over to her good friend and hair specialist Krista Bradford. Krista demonstrates how to create this intricate voluminous curled bun effect using just a curling iron, tail comb, bobby pins, a hair tie and hairspray. As Michelle would say, the result sure is one "prettyful" look and it works well on both her dark mane and Krista's light blonde locks.

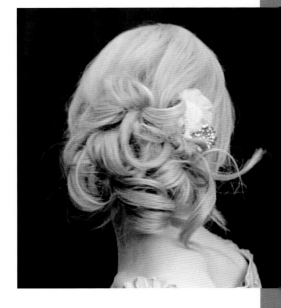

Summer Hair Trend: Top Knot

Catwalk chic with
Makeup Geek

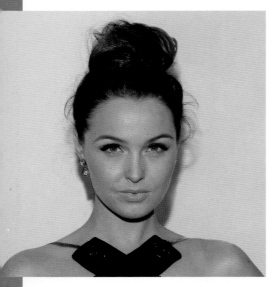

The top-knot bun is one of a few catwalk staple looks that is actually really easy to recreate, which is why it's been quick to take off among fashionistas all over the world, including Sienna Miller, Kate Bosworth and Nicole Richie. This bold style works on any type or length of hair, whether it's clean or dirty, making it a saviour on bad hair days. Watch as Paige, the hair guru from beauty blog Makeup Geek, demonstrates just how simple it is to achieve this polished and interesting look, even when you have only a few minutes to spare.

http://youtu.be/PzvmwWORj6k

Braided Bun Updo

Recycle old socks with Bebexo

Been thinking about buying one of those hair donuts to help you create a full, thick-looking bun? Well, you might want to postpone that particular shopping trip until you've watched this clip from Nee, aka beauty blogger Bebexo. Nee has discovered a way to turn an old sock into a hair donut in just two simple steps – well, three, as you'll probably want to wash the sock first! Nee has also created an unusual way to add braids to your bun for a unique textured look – no wonder the clip has been viewed more than 5 million times. So what are you waiting for? Get raiding that sock drawer!

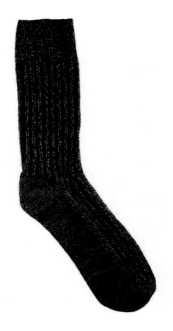

http://youtu.be/9farzQTWOC8

Easy No-Heat Up Styles

RachhLoves makes high-fashion hair look easy

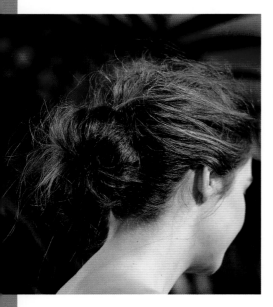

Canadian YouTube star RachhLoves is a big fan of trying out new hairdos, paying special attention to low-effort techniques that deliver maximum style. Her top styling tips start by making your own sea-salt water spray and spritzing your hair with it the night before for maximum texture. She then applies a curling mousse just to the bottom half of her hair before twisting up into a bun to sleep in. Next morning you run baby powder or dry shampoo through your hair for extra volume and you're ready to style. Rachel then demos two pretty but messy updos – both made in 5 minutes just by twisting and adding a few pins. Hair magic.

http://youtu.be/dom_ElqLpYc

Sparkly Chignon

The Beauty Department's bejewelled party hair

TV star Lauren Conrad's one-stop shop for all things hair is a fabulous place to find updo inspiration. The pictures are always stunning and the steps are oh-so-simple to follow. In this video, hair ends are curled before an elastic jewelled hairband is added, into which hair is twisted up and back, and then tucked into the headband. The end result is a gorgeous style that would work equally well for a night at the pub or for a more glam party – all in less than 2 minutes. A fantastic tutorial, which exemplifies why beauty vlogging is the perfect medium for teaching anyone how to create gorgeous hair.

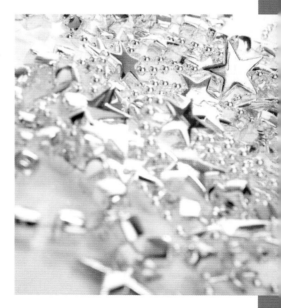

http://youtu.be/4bBblo-8x90

Quick Half Updo

Get some root volume with Dulce Tejeda

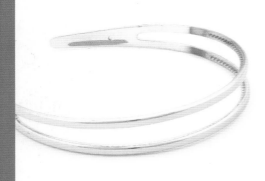

The main problem with Dulce Tejeda's YouTube channel, DulceCandy87, is that you can't just watch one video. The addictive beauty savvy vlogger has a range of informative makeup and hair tutorials, all delivered in an adorably cute style. Little wonder she's become the go-to blogger for 1.7 million subscribers. Here she shows how to create a simple half-up half-down do. She straightens her hair first with irons, then backcombs the crown and adds a little hairspray for volume, before pinning it back and adding a hair band. Her top tip for keeping a wayward fringe (bangs) right where you want it, is to spray it with hairspray and pin it in place until it dries – after which you can remove the pin.

http://youtu.be/A8yg6BDGWsl

Messy Side Bun

Effortless sophistication with
Emma Pickles

British vlogger Emma Pickles' Euphoric Creations
videos regularly get over a million views and with
their amazing creative designs and clever celeb
copies it's easy to see why. Emma's top updo tips
include only attempting them at least two days
after washing hair to maximize grip, and adding
some loose curls at the bottom of locks using a hair
straightener before using the same tool to straighten
the roots for a smooth finish once up. For this look,
hair is pulled into a low side ponytail and then
pieces are backcombed and tucked and pinned into
the hairband, all the way around. But don't be too
precise, as "Messy is good" says Emma. Finally she
curls her fringe (bangs) backwards for a model finish
– proving it's the little details that count.

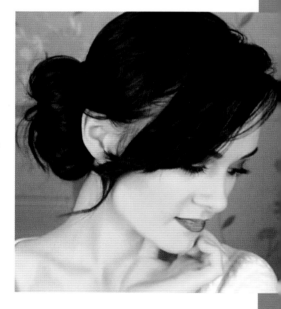

Two-Minute Hair Tuck

Essie Button rocks
festival chic

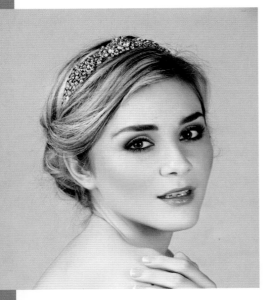

Essie Button is the vlogging alias of Canadian blogger Estée, who lives in London. Her channel is one of the best around for easy but effective hair how-tos, particularly for fine hair. In this video Estée demos her ridiculously simple updo technique. She adds a bit of Alberto VO5 Instant Oomph Hair Powder and works it into the roots around the crown, then puts on a pretty hairband. Sides are tucked into the band and the back gathered in a ponytail and tucked in too. Top tips are to pull extra pieces of the hair out to create a more messy, natural look. Perfect for festivals as you can do this style pretty much anywhere or on-the-go.

http://youtu.be/n2Tqany08T4

Speedy Twisted Updo

Bubzbeauty beats a "bad hair"
day in minutes

It's the morning after the night before, and not only
have you woken up with a head full of frizz, but you
also have minutes to get ready to leave the house
– argh! But before you reach for the bobble hat, all
is not lost, as Lindy Tsang of Bubzbeauty is here to
show you how to transform bed head into an
elegant and romantic twisted updo in just 3 minutes.
This simple style suits straight, curly or wavy hair
and both Taylor Swift and Gwen Stefani have been
spotted out with it. And if it's good enough for
them… count us in.

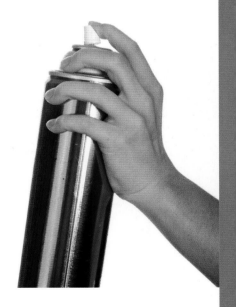

http://youtu.be/Bf-gRNE0uDs

Messy Twisted Bun

RachhLoves' refreshing style
for day-old hair

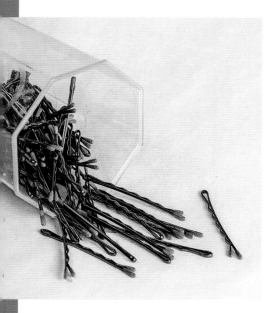

Transform hair that's a little stale into a cute stylish updo, in less time than it takes to make a cup of tea. Perfect after a day at the beach, or if you've just been invited on a spontaneous night out and there's not enough time to wash and style before you have to go. Canadian girl Rachel adores the sun, sea and sand, so she has plenty of experience dealing with windswept hair. In this popular clip she reveals her 2-minute trick for creating a cute, twisted updo with just a hair band and a couple of pins.

http://youtu.be/_ItHsbsG7Ao

Posh Plaited Bun

Take a bun to a whole new level with Pixiwoo

Buns are a perennial favourite updo for vintage glamour. Perfect for a day at the races, a friend's wedding or an awards ceremony. But if you want to stand out from the crowd, rather than blend into the sea of smooth buns, then this is the bun for you. Sam Chapman, one half of beauty duo Pixiwoo, is here to show you how to not only create a fishtail plait (braid) in 5 minutes, but also how to then pin it into a beautiful bun. Don't miss Sam's tip for recycling old jewellery into a glitzy hair accessory. Now that's what we call vintage!

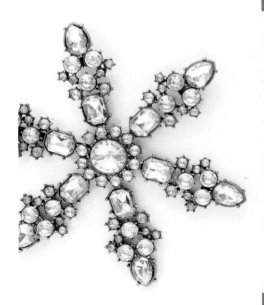

http://youtu.be/kxl4BECWedI

Half-Up Cute Hair

Luxy Hair's easy trick for
sculpting hair into a bow

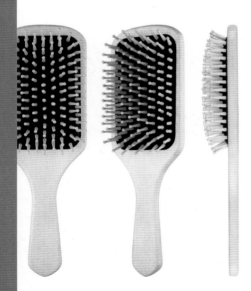

Why wear a bow to fasten your hair, when your hair can be the bow? Mimi from Luxy Hair admits that for a long time she was intimidated by this complicated-looking hairstyle. But when she decided to revisit it, she discovered a simple technique for creating this beautiful look in minutes. As Mimi says, "It just goes to show you sometimes you have to try things a few times to get it." All you need to create your hair bow is a brush, hair pins, one elastic hairband and two mirrors – so you can see what you're doing at the back of your head as you work.

http://youtu.be/94sY1i39fho

Easy Updo for Long Hair

Free your neck with
Emma Pickles' tutorial

Really thick, long hair can seem like more of a burden than a blessing on hot days when it just won't behave. There's just no easy way to pull your hair up off your neck – as even when tied up it generally still covers the back of your neck in an uncomfortable, thick layer. Emma Pickles does not have ultra-long hair, but in the spirit of friendship she's donned extensions in order to help her longer-maned viewers overcome this conundrum. Follow this short and simple tutorial to learn how to create a cute style that not only lifts all hair off your neck, but is finished off with a patterned scarf for a cute retro look.

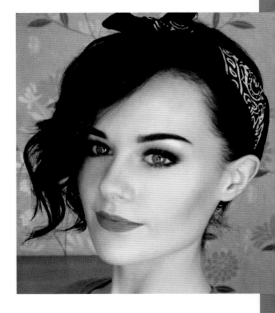

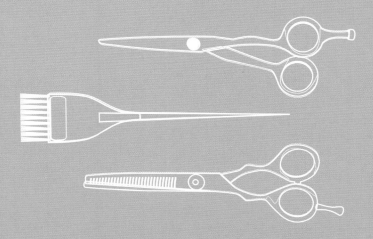

AT-HOME

Haircare

How to Wash Curly Hair

Lock in the moisture and banish frizz with Whitney White

Natural hair guru Whitney White, aka Naptural85, has invaluable tips on caring for textured hair – including lots of amazing DIY product recipes. Washing naturally very curly hair isn't always easy, but here Whitney takes you through her failsafe technique, starting with a top tip of making sure you haven't got any chipped nails or jagged edges, which can catch and snap hair. She then splits hair into sections and applies her DIY cider vinegar and water mix, which works as a clarifier to breakdown oil and product build up, before massaging her homemade mayonnaise deep conditioner all over. Watch out for another useful tip on using oil to seal in moisture post-conditioner.

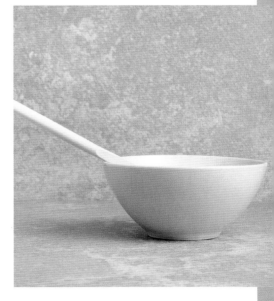

Salon Deep Treatment at Home

Kasey Palmer's DIY
conditioning mask

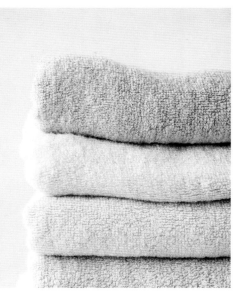

Kasey Palmer is a vlogging pro, whose direct delivery and expert hair and makeup advice hit the mark every time. In this popular clip she shows how to do your own deep conditioning hair treatment – the kind you would fork out lots of money for at the salon. She uses pure vitamin E oil mixed with ordinary intensive conditioner, but advises it's worth investing in a really good one. The mixture is then massaged into dry – not wet – hair, so your locks can really absorb all of the moisture, and then wrapped in a hot towel for 20 minutes. Kasey recommends a final rinse in cold water to close hair cuticles for added shine.

http://youtu.be/sZ4OQF22bBY

Caring for Ombre Hair

Boost your blonde
bits with Zoella

Makeup and hair guru Zoe Sugg's exuberant personality and beauty know-how has attracted 5.5 million subscribers to her beauty channel Zoella, confirming her as YouTube royalty. Here the bubbly Brit shares how she cares for her ombre hair – which is bleached from midway down to the tips, leaving the ends fragile and dry. This useful guide is perfect for anyone who has joined the ombre hair craze and needs tips on keeping their hair in decent condition. Top tips include only using shampoos for coloured hair and in particular, investing in a "purple" shampoo that tones blonde hair colours and helps eradicate any brassy, yellow tones.

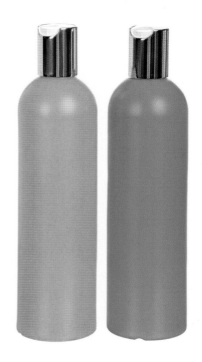

http://youtu.be/mMHK6F5TRBc

Homemade Remedies for Frizzy Hair

AndreasChoice keeps
your curls in check

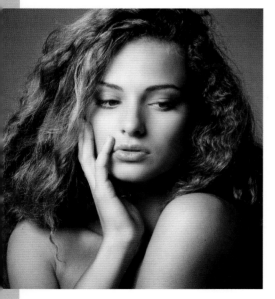

Andrea Brooks of AndreasChoice is full of great DIY beauty tips and tricks. In a clip that has been viewed more than a million times she outlines three deep treatments you can make for yourself. The first uses lime juice and coconut milk, which Andrea explains are great for your hair because when combined they help control unruly locks. The next conditioner combines honey and yoghurt and the third mixes your own standard conditioner with olive oil. Whichever mixture you pick, Andrea says the trick is to leave it on as long as possible – ideally overnight –before rinsing off. Other top taming tips include never towelling dry hair, and rewetting it a second time to help "clump" hair together so it's less likely to frizz when fully dried.

http://youtu.be/Cq4GUFBRnhM

Looking after Long Hair

Protect lengthier locks
with Fleur DeForce

Keeping long hair in superb condition isn't easy, as the longer it is, the older it is, and therefore the more damage it's likely to have suffered. Here British vlogger Fleur DeForce name-checks her favourite shampoo for long locks, pointing out that you don't need to spend a fortune to find a decent one. She does suggest always using a leave-in conditioner to detangle hair and make it easier to comb though while wet, and also recommends finding a good once-a-week deep conditioner. Other top tips include using a paddle brush, which doesn't snag on long hair, and ignoring high-end heat protectors in favour of a budget version, as Fleur hasn't found there's any difference in performance.

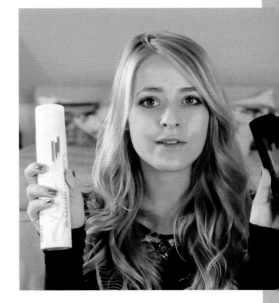

Get More Beautiful Hair

Cassandra Bankson shares
her softer hair secrets

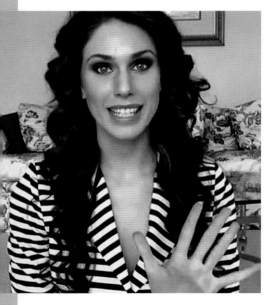

Looking for the lowdown on simple everyday hair care that will make your hair soft, shiny and thick? Cassandra Bankson spills the secrets behind her luscious locks on her DiamondsAndHeels14 channel, and the best thing is, the US model's routine doesn't involve any expensive products or difficult-to-master techniques. Instead she shares easy-to-follow steps that can be worked into your daily routine, including her favourite hair oil – which you can pick up in health food stores not pricey salons. She also offers her advice on what to look for in a shampoo, including avoiding "sulphates" because, Cassandra says, they strip hair of its natural oils, leaving it dry and damaged.

http://youtu.be/clFJtr8QpAU

Make Your Own Deep Conditioner

Save a bundle with
MissGlamorazzi's product recipe

MissGlamorazzi, aka Ingrid Nilsen, discovered the importance of a good conditioner at a young age. She was a swimmer in high school and her hair would get really dried out by the chlorine. So she set about perfecting a recipe for the best homemade deep conditioner, using ingredients from her kitchen. After a bit of trial and error she hit on this recipe using just three nourishing ingredients – avocado, olive oil and honey – and it produced such good results that she's been using it ever since. If you want hair as soft, shiny and healthy as Ingrid's without an expensive salon treatment every week, then watch this clip and give it a try.

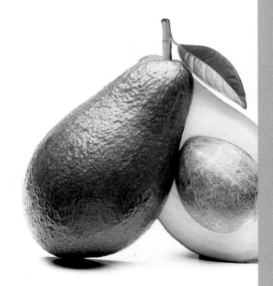

No Time to Wash Your Hair?

Blair Fowler's expert guide to dry shampoo

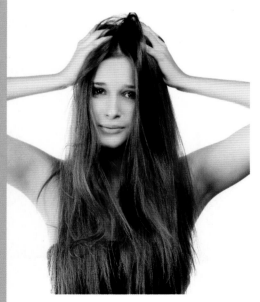

Fast-talking Blair is so dedicated to finding the very best hair products that she's spent weeks testing various dry shampoos to find one that doesn't give dark hair an unfortunate grey tinge. Think of Blair as your human guinea pig; she's done the hard work, so you don't have to. In this vlog on her Juicystar07 channel the younger Fowler sister reveals her top dry shampoo pick, and the good news is it's made by Lush, so you can pick it up on the high street. The product is a powder rather than a spray, but while it may look a little odd at first, Blair promises once you've tried it you'll never go back to dry shampoo spray again.

http://youtu.be/ri8WBOmd_8s

Treat Split Ends

Tanya Burr's pick of the best smoothing products

Unfortunately split ends are a fact of life. They are as inevitable as the latest celebrity scandal and the only way to get rid of them is to cut them off. But in between trips to the hairdressers, there are some products that can keep split ends at bay for a little longer than usual, and others that will improve the appearance of hair that has already started to split. Watch this vlog to discover the affordable TRESemmé and Dove products that makeup artist Tanya Burr swears by to keep the ends of her hair in tip-top condition, from shampoo to leave-in treatment and even the best 60-second fix.

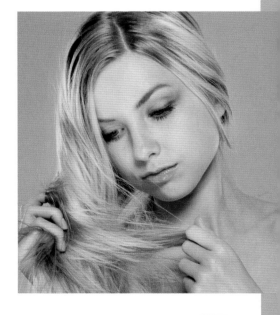

http://youtu.be/_RfRnBW9eq4

Cut Your Own Fringe at Home

Avoid the hairdresser with Julia Graf's cutting technique

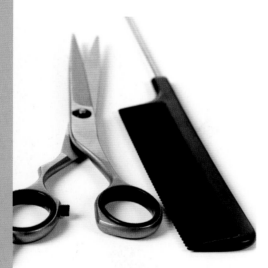

Hate getting your fringe (bangs) cut in at the hairdressers, because they never quite understand how you want it? Julia Graf can relate, as she always steps out of the salon with side-swept bangs that bear no resemblance to the choppy fringe she was after. After the last salon disappointment she had an epiphany – "You know what, life's short," she declares. "Don't waste your time worrying about your hair. It's going to grow back." In this clip on her MissChievous channel, Swiss makeup artist Julia demonstrates using her own hair just how easy it is to create a "piecey" fringe at home. Don't be scared of the scissors – you can do it!

http://youtu.be/WdgVo9BWkyQ

Grow Longer Hair, Fast

The tricks behind Cassandra Bankson's long locks

The length of Cassandra Bankson's hair is truly impressive. It falls in thick curly waves that reach halfway down her back. But before you switch off, overcome with jealousy, bear in mind that everything Californian-girl Cassandra does to make her hair grow long, thick and strong is easily achievable. In this vlog the professional model spills all her secrets, and there isn't an expensive hair growth elixir in sight, just some tried and tested advice that can be easily worked into your daily routine to give your hair a natural boost. Top tips include using products containing scalp-stimulating essential oils such as peppermint or tea tree oil and identifying the right foods for healthy hair.

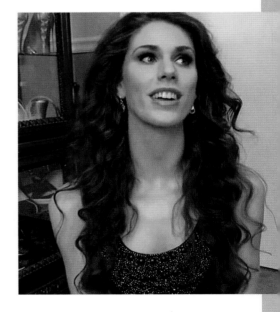

http://youtu.be/BawaBZfIjUE

How to Cut Layers in Your Hair

Be your own hairdresser
with Carlibel55

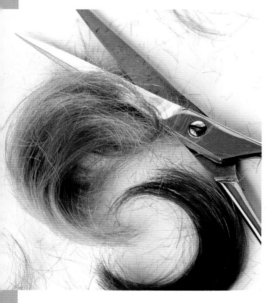

This vlog comes with a word of warning: Carli of popular YouTube channel the Beauty Bybel is not a trained hairdresser, however she has been chopping her own hair for years and she's developed an effective cutting style for creating her long layers. "I'm not saying my way is right, so try it at your own risk," Carli cautions. The vlogger is certainly confident, hacking away long lengths at a time as she talks, demonstrating her technique step-by-step on her own hair, although she advises that you "just do a little bit at a time" so it's easier to correct any mistakes. The results are impressive but if you're not feeling brave enough, you can always take a screenshot of Carli's hair to your hairdresser!

http://youtu.be/SHl3Wi4ghQk

DIY Hair Growth Treatment

The scalp secrets behind AndreasChoice's long locks

Healthy strong hair can grow up to 15cm (6in) a year, but unfortunately for most of us our hair falls short of this sort of growth. Why? Because we've not taken proper care of our scalp, says vlogger Andrea Brooks of AndreasChoice. There are many expensive treatments available which promise to promote hair growth by stimulating blood flow to the scalp, but before you splash the cash you may want to join the many thousands of viewers who have checked out this vlog, in which Andrea reveals the unlikely "badass" store cupboard staple behind her healthy scalp – an onion. Andrea uses the pungent veg to create a sulphur-rich on-scalp treatment to help feed follicles and promote new hair growth.

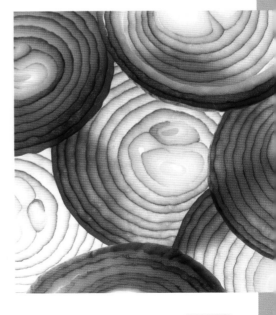

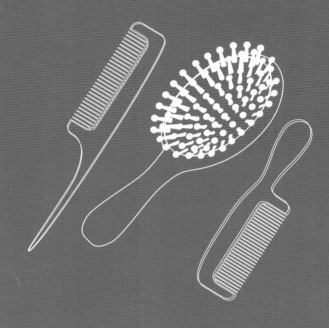

GET THE

Look

Brigitte Bardot Hair Tutorial

Luxy Hair's subtle sex symbol styling

Mimi from Luxy Hair is a big fan of Brigitte Bardot's bed-head bouffant. "She's such a classic beauty and she's been such an inspiration to me," says Mimi of the actress, "she's somebody who is effortless and sexy at the same time." Unsurprisingly, Mimi loves to recreate the sixties sex symbol's iconic wavy half-updo, not least because it's disarmingly simple. Learn how easy this look is to create with just a curling iron, bobby pins and a teasing brush. Indeed, simplicity is in fact the key to achieving Brigitte's look. "Her look was never overdone," Mimi adds. "It was almost like she just rolled out of bed and she looked so sexy and beautiful."

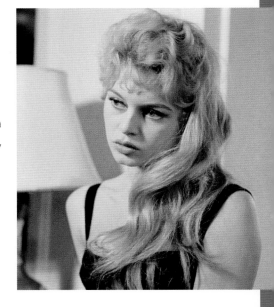

http://youtu.be/c4BdEOaxFEw

Four Summer Hairstyles in Minutes

Bubzbeauty's lovely low-maintenance looks

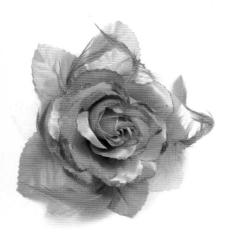

Looking for a new go-to style that you can easily adapt to suit different days? Once you've mastered the styling in this vlog, you'll be able to create a look for any occasion. Rather than taking you through four separate styles, Lindy Tsang, aka Bubzbeauty, creates four looks that develop from one to another. Starting with a cute and girly half updo that only takes 2 minutes, the Irish blogger then works through an elegant and sweet side style, explains how to add an extra touch of elegance by styling your fringe (bangs), before finally transforming the look into a soft princess look with the help of a curling wand.

http://youtu.be/2yVpTaiEl5o

Three Easy Date-Night Hairstyles

Make him swoon with
MissGlamorazzi's romantic styles

In this 8-minute clip from MissGlamorazzi, you'll learn all the styling secrets you need to create perfect date night hair – not just for your first date, but also for the second and the third that will surely follow when your hair looks this good! Each style is totally different so you'll keep your date intrigued. The first style is a glam updo paired with a red lip. Look two is ultra feminine soft and girly curls, perfect for a daytime date, while look three is a classic chic chignon that will showcase your sophisticated side. Little wonder around 700,000 people have viewed this very useful video.

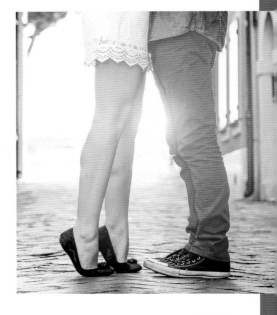

http://youtu.be/ynHDLo5mjfM

1960s Beehive

Ruth Crilly adds a modern edge to a classic look

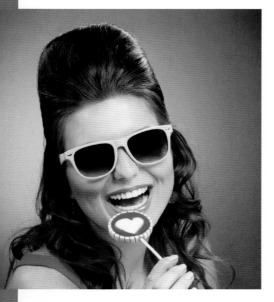

Beehives were big business in the 1960s, and while they are still an eye-catching look, wearing your hair in a full "hive" can make you feel as if you're going to a retro-themed party. But fashion model Ruth Crilly's clever twist on this classic look brings it bang up-to-date. Her half-up-half-down beehive gives you all the gorgeous height and volume of the original look, but with a more relaxed contemporary softness to it. In this clip from her popular A Model Recommends channel, don't miss Ruth's technique for creating volume that will give roots a lift, while keeping the hair smooth on top.

http://youtu.be/Jkq56uhUE2M

We Found Love-Inspired Hair Tutorial

Beautycrush channels Rihanna's cool curls

Fashion graduate Sammi Maria's vlogs usually focus on fashion, but she's been inspired to step out of her comfort zone by some impressive hair styling she spotted in a pop video. In *We Found Love* Rihanna sports ringlets, which she scoops into a pretty updo secured by a bandana, and Sammi certainly shares the love she's found for this style with her step-by-step clip explaining exactly how you can create this edgy, carefree look. Particularly useful is Sammi's tips on how to use straighteners to create defined curls just at the ends of your hair.

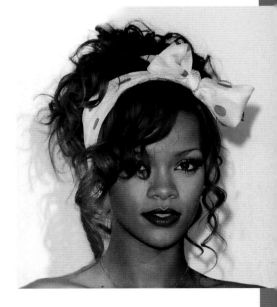

Taylor Swift Soft Waves

Get country-girl cute
with Julia Graf

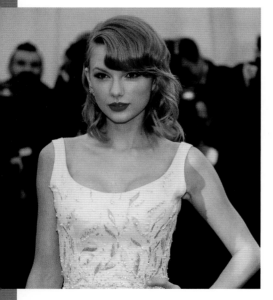

Think of Taylor Swift and the first thing that comes to mind (well okay, the second, after that infamous incident with Kanye West at the VMAs) is her signature hairstyle: soft blonde waves and chunky, blunt fringe (bangs). In this vlog, Swiss-Candian hair and makeup guru Julia Graf demonstrates how to recreate Taylor's iconic "soft, sleek, sexy and sultry" look, including how to give your fringe bouncy volume and how to use a large barrel roller to create long-lasting flowing waves instead of ringlets. Julia proves this is a look that suits everyone, not just pop stars. So what are you waiting for? Give yourself the hairstyle that once bagged One Direction's Harry Styles…

http://youtu.be/TnPtYLctVTl

Quick Daytime Styles

Go back to beauty school with Bethany Mota

Add four new style strings to your bow with this one brief beauty tuition session from YouTube megastar Bethany Mota. All four styles are easy and quick to create, making them perfect looks for school for the American vlogger's millions of teenage "Mota-vator" fans. But don't be put off if your school days are well and truly behind you, these looks translate well into the working world too. What's more they don't involve any heat styling, so they won't damage your hair. Learn how to create an intricate three braids in one style, a pretty bow updo, a braided headband crafted from your fringe (bangs) and a "unique and cool" side-swept fishtail plait (braid).

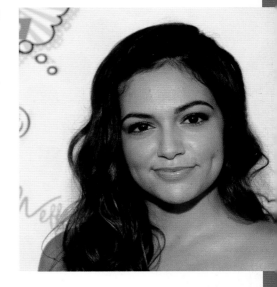

Elsa from *Frozen*'s Volumized Braid

Let It Go! with a pretty princess plait
by Foxy Locks

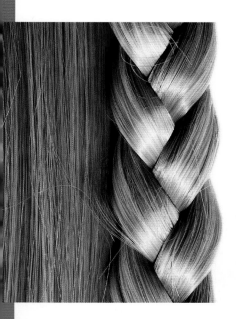

Dresses based on the costume worn by Elsa in the Disney film *Frozen* (the highest grossing animated film of all time) sell out as soon as they hit shop floors. If you're a little old to be picking up clothes from the Disney Store but still fancy emulating an ice princess look, a more subtle and sophisticated approach is to learn how to craft Elsa's signature volumized French plait (braid) hairstyle. Imogen of specialist hair channel Foxy Locks is just the girl to show you how to master the tricky combination of volume at the roots and a long French plait in this simple step-by-step tutorial.

http://youtu.be/jibusAsAH5g

Five Quick and Easy Styles

Zoella's speedy styling
for pretty perfection

Zoe Sugg's long thick locks are always styled to perfection in her vlogs. Whether it's in a high ponytail, a chunky braid or loose waves, she never has a hair out of place. You'd be forgiven for thinking that she spends hours styling her mane before every take, but you'd be wrong. "In all honesty it doesn't take me very long," says Zoe. "I am not one of these people who spends a lot of time on my hair." Learn how you can create the five fast styles that Britain's biggest beauty blogger (with more than 5 million subscribers) has in her hair arsenal. Top tip: watch right to the end for an extra comedy style!

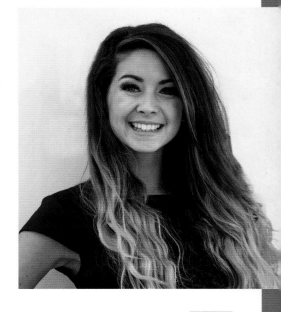

Hollywood Glamour Tutorial

Hannah Leigh's hairstyle is guaranteed to make waves

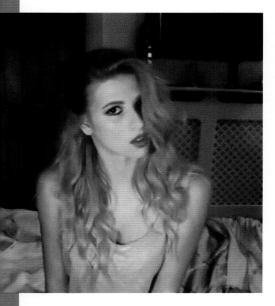

Nothing screams Hollywood film star quite like big glossy waves. It can be tricky either to tame curls or to tease straight hair into this polished look, which is why for many years it's been the domain solely of the celebrity stylist. But Sheffield-born Hannah Leigh has perfected a curling and combing technique, which makes it easy to achieve this Hollywood-standard style at home. All you need is a curling iron, brush and hairspray and heat protecting spray. Finish off the look with a splash of bold lip colour and a flick of smoky eyes, to fully embody the aura of an actress straight from the silver screen.

http://youtu.be/VGpN6KRP0cw?list

Fauxhawk Mohawk Tutorial

Bring out your inner rock chick
with Julia Graf

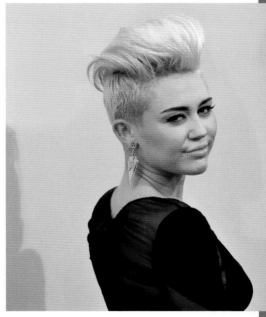

This striking look is not for the fainthearted, but if you want a style that will make you stand out among the crowd and you're not afraid of using half a ton of hairspray to achieve it, then this is the vlog for you. Swiss-based YouTube star Julia Graf demonstrates how to create a faux mohawk, without shaving the sides of your head. She crafts her locks into a voluminous bouffant on top with slicked-back sides using lots of backcombing and hairspray. Be warned: normal hairspray will not pass muster for this "rock hard" look, so don't miss Julia's advice on picking the right type to keep your hair high all night.

Pixie Lott / Lauren Conrad Hair

The style that's making waves from London to LA

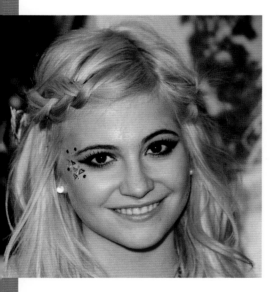

The Hills' star Lauren Conrad and London-based pop princess Pixie Lott share a love of styling their long blonde locks in a laidback boho fashion. When asked about her favourite hair-do Pixie said, "I love experimenting with styles like little plaits," while Californian Lauren has revealed that it often takes her 7 hours to fit her hair extensions! Well, Lauren and Pixie may both want to tune into this vlog from Hannah Leigh, as the Sheffield chameleon demonstrates how to complete the duo's most celebrated hairstyle – complete with both little plaits (braids) and hair extensions – in under 4 minutes.

http://youtu.be/vmewVdDl6qM?list

Six Lazy Styles

AndreasChoice's go-to styles
for busy mornings

Are you guilty of wearing your hair in the same style every day? When time is tight in the mornings it can be easy to rely on one easy look that's smart enough to pass muster. But Andrea's here to show you six funky alternative styles that will keep your hair out of your face all day long and best of all they're super-quick to achieve. Andrea admits that she's having a bad hair day while filming this tutorial, which just goes to show that each of these looks is capable of transforming the worst of hair days into an excuse to show off a new sleek style.

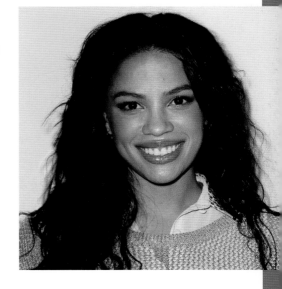

Rihanna's Grammys Hair

Aim for award-winning style with Jenny Strebe

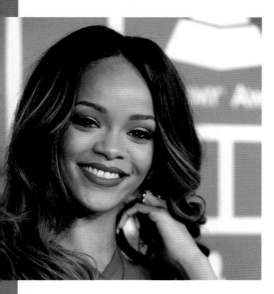

Even beauty newbies can score unique, salon-worthy locks at home with hairstylist turned vlogger Jenny Strebe's easy-to-follow tutorials on Confessions of a Hairstylist. An avid believer that updos (and all hairstyles for that matter) should be totally uncomplicated and definitely not stiff, Jenny is the perfect guide to recreate the voluminous curls worn by Rihanna at the 2013 Grammys. This stunning look is easy to achieve with just a curling wand and some bobby pins, and can be worn by any hair type or length.

http://youtu.be/7yuFPCEG22I?list

Pretty Little Liars Look

RachhLoves' take on Hanna Marin's long-lasting waves

Hanna Marin, the character played by actress Ashley Benson in *Pretty Little Liars*, is so hot right now. Her girly yet edgy style is always ahead of the curve and just like any good trendsetter she's always changing her hairstyle. One of Hanna's most striking looks is when she wears her hair in soft beachy waves. You can achieve the same natural finish and non-uniform curls by following this fun tutorial from RachhLoves using a cone-shaped curling wand. A common problem with curls is that they tend to fall out throughout the course of the day, but lifestyle vlogger Rachel knows a trick or two to give this look real staying power.

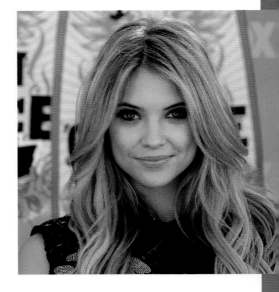

Do a Dita Von Teese

Pin-up appeal in 10 minutes
with Pixiwoo

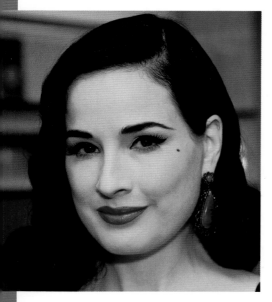

Want to create a sultry style worthy of the burlesque queen in just 10 minutes? Well, Sam from British beauty vlogging duo Pixiwoo has mastered the art of the instant bombshell wave and she's here to show you how you can too. "I call this my easy Dita Von Teese style," she says. "And it is easy. It's not of course how she does her hair – it takes a lot more time to do her hair than this. But not all of us have the time or the level of skill of her hairdresser, so we'll just do it the easy way." Hear! Hear!

http://youtu.be/J4M3I6-1jMk

Bridesmaid Braid for Long Hair

Perfect "Disney Princess" hair
with Zoella

Certain occasions call for an attention-grabbing look, and this sideways waterfall plaiting (braiding) technique, from Britain's biggest beauty vlogger, will certainly have people marvelling at your mane. This is not your everyday run-of-the mill plait. Zoella explains it requires time, practice and – unless you are a very skilled hairstyler – the help of a friend (or indeed a fellow bridesmaid). But this gorgeously romantic look is well worth the effort. The pretty flower-decorated braid appears to defy gravity as it drapes through the middle of your glossy, bouncing curls. Remember, practice makes perfect, so watch this vlog a few times before the big day.

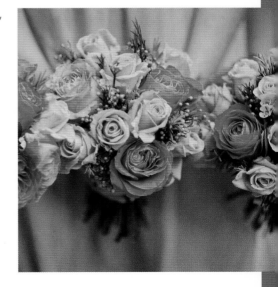

Running Late Looks

Luxy Hair demos three
hairstyles in 3 minutes!

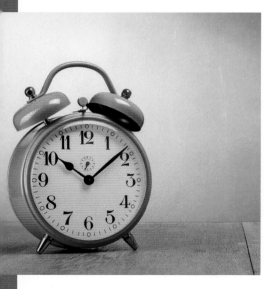

We've all been there, those mornings when you sleep through your alarm and wake up with only 5 minutes before you're due to leave the house. Just thinking about it is enough to make you panic, which is why this vlog tutorial, for three hairstyles that take 60 seconds each to create, has been viewed more than 6 million times! Mimi from Luxy Hair shows three ways of styling your hair so that no one will ever be able to tell you rushed through your morning routine. All you need is hair pins, hair bands, hairspray, a teasing comb, a hair donut – and 1 minute to spare.

http://youtu.be/zugLQF3uLmk

Five No-Heat Summer Styles

Say bye-bye to overheated hair
with Bethany Mota

On hot days the last thing you want to do is spend hours with your hair using heated tools, which is why YouTube superstar Bethany Mota has created this collection of five fun and funky styles that can be achieved with no heat at all. There's something for everyone here, whatever your level of hair styling skill, and no matter how much (or how little) time you have to spare. Learn how to create a messy fishtail with twists, a French braided side bun, a girly braided updo and two reversible braids that work for both formal and more relaxed events.

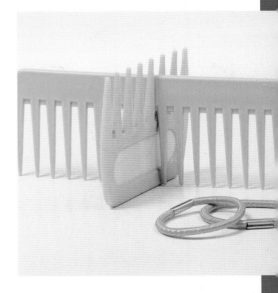

http://youtu.be/mGaN41UDQvs

Kim Kardashian's Signature Hair

Get Kim K's cute curls
with Jessica Harlow

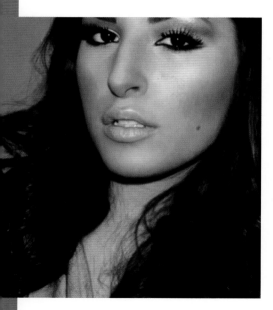

Kim Kardashian's second most famous asset is her flowing dark locks, which are always styled to polished perfection. Beauty vlogger Jessica Harlow is a big fan of KK's hair, especially her signature sexy curls that start from half way down the head. "It's classic without being boring," says fellow brunette blogger. "You can wear this kind of hair style anywhere, especially to any kind of special event where your photo will be taken, and years from now you can look back without any embarrassment." With Jessica's expert help, the look that drives the paparazzi crazy is super easy to achieve, as nearly 400,000 views for this clip proves.

http://youtu.be/AWISN1YWwcc

Victoria's Secret Hair

Kasey Palmer's tricks for creating
a sex-bomb barnet

Victoria's Secret models do not need eye-catching hair – their amazing scantily clad bodies are grabbing enough attention already. But nonetheless, the hairstylists behind the scenes at every catwalk show rise to the challenge of creating hairstyles that vie for attention with the lingerie. The supermodel's signature style is big voluminous sex-kitten loose curls, a look that has the power to transform anyone into a bombshell. Vlogger Kasey Palmer is here to show how everyone from tired mums to shrinking violets can recreate the look, plus the Southern American also demonstrates how to seamlessly (and secretly) blend hair extensions into your natural hair if you need added length to get the full VS "angels" look.

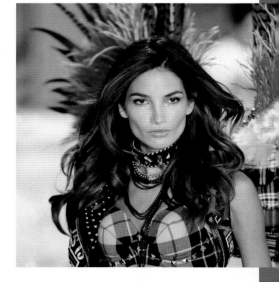

http://youtu.be/u2su8d4GJO8

Great Gatsby Faux Bob

Toni & Guy's approved technique
for faking a bob

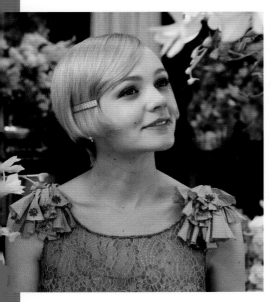

The recent remake of *The Great Gatsby* showcased a flamboyant 1920s style that had a rush of people hankering after angular flapper-style bobs. However, when it comes to the crunch (or should that be the cut) many women with longer hair chicken out at the last minute. But long-locked ladies don't need to miss out on this vintage glamour style. In this clip Toni & Guy's award-winning hair stylist Darian shares her secrets for shaping longer hair in such a way that it looks like it's been lopped off just below the jawline. This is not an easy look to master, but the more ambitious and skilled home stylists will certainly benefit from Darian's salon-schooled expertise.

http://youtu.be/klix2iF9wFA

Go Vintage with Faux Victory Rolls

Cherry Dollface's easy take on classic 1940s glamour

Twisting hair into "victory rolls" was first popularized in the 1940s when the style was worn at parties to celebrate the end of the Second World War. Now they've become a great statement style for a vintage dance party, rockabilly night out, or simply when you want to inject some old skool glamour into an otherwise modern look. The only problem is, true victory rolls are every bit as tricky to perfect as they look! But if you're worried your styling skills aren't quite up to the challenge, fear not, Californian vlogger of all things vintage, Cherry Dollface, is here to reveal how to create the illusion of a victory roll, with this easy-to-master faux style. Hurray!

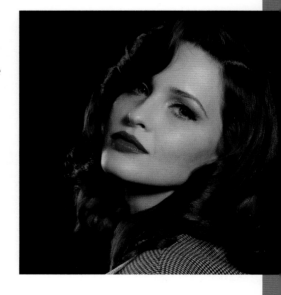

http://youtu.be/pzaNNhHbCJ0

The Author

Caroline Jones is a beauty, fashion and health journalist who has been a senior editor on several national newspapers and magazines in the UK. She is the author of five books, including *The Busy Girl's Guide to Looking Great* and *1001 Ways to Spend Less and Look Beautiful*. Caroline lives in London with her daughter and husband.

Picture Credits